Understanding Hepatotoxicity - Causes, Symptoms and Prevention

Edited by Xingshun Qi and Xiaofeng Liu

Published in London, United Kingdom

Understanding Hepatotoxicity - Causes, Symptoms and Prevention
http://dx.doi.org/10.5772/intechopen.1005942
Edited by Xingshun Qi and Xiaofeng Liu

Contributors
Chenghai Liu, Eduardo Pena, Fei Gao, Haijuan Lv, Hongwei Zhao, Huikuan Chu, Hu Liu, Marco Luza, Qianqian Li, Qinke Wu, Sam Johnson Udhayachandar, Ting Wang, Vignesh Pandi, Xiaofeng Liu, Xingshun Qi, Ye Yang

First published in London, United Kingdom, 2025 by IntechOpen
IntechOpen is the global imprint of INTECHOPEN LIMITED, registered in England and Wales, registration number: 11086078, 167-169 Great Portland Street, London, W1W 5PF, United Kingdom

For EU product safety concerns: IN TECH d.o.o., Prolaz Marije Krucifikse Kozulić 3, 51000 Rijeka, Croatia, info@intechopen.com or visit our website at intechopen.com.

British Library Cataloguing-in-Publication Data
A catalogue record for this book is available from the British Library

Understanding Hepatotoxicity - Causes, Symptoms and Prevention
Edited by Xingshun Qi and Xiaofeng Liu
p. cm.
Print ISBN 978-1-83634-560-2
Online ISBN 978-1-83634-559-6
eBook (PDF) ISBN 978-1-83634-561-9

Meet the editor

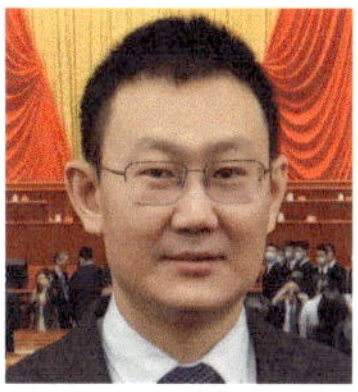

Dr. Xingshun Qi is the head of the Department of Gastroenterology of the General Hospital of Northern Theater Command, China. His primary research interests are in clinical research related to the etiology, diagnosis, and management of liver cirrhosis, portal hypertension, portal vein thrombosis, Budd-Chiari syndrome, and hepatocellular carcinoma. He serves as a senior editorial board member of BMC Gastroenterology, an editorial board member of Advances in Therapy and Therapeutic Advances in Gastroenterology, and an academic editor of the Canadian Journal of Gastroenterology and Hepatology and the Journal of Clinical and Translational Hepatology. His H-index is 53 now.

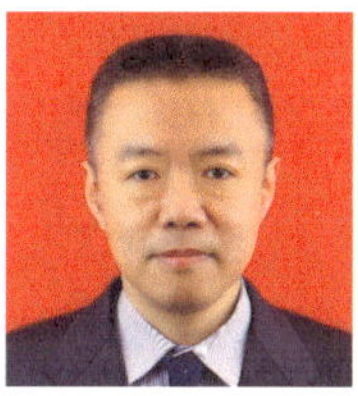

Prof. Dr. Xiaofeng Liu is the Director of the Department of Gastroenterology of the 960th Hospital of the PLA. Currently, he is a member of the Gastroenterology Branch of the Chinese Medical Association and the chairman of the Hepatology Branch of the Shandong Provincial Medical Doctor Association. He is skilled in the management of digestive system diseases, with a great specialty in managing complex cases of cirrhotic portal hypertension and advancing the understanding of gastrointestinal cancers through bench-to-bedside research. He has published over 60 articles in both Chinese and English as the first or corresponding author, edited one book as chief editor, and completed seven monographs. He has received multiple national and provincial scientific research funds and medical achievement awards.

Contents

Preface

The liver is the central organ of metabolism in the human body and is responsible for removing toxic substances. When excessive toxins, including various chemical drugs, enter the liver, it will be overburdened, thereby being injured and disabled, even developing liver failure and death, which is referred to as hepatotoxicity. Nowadays, it has been shown that lots of drugs, such as antibiotics, herbal medications, traditional Chinese medicine, and immune checkpoint inhibitors, can cause hepatic damage, which is characterized by elevated levels of transaminase, alkaline phosphatase, and gamma-glutamyltransferase. This unexpected phenomenon is often termed as drug-induced liver injury. Clinicians and patients must have access to current knowledge regarding the management of hepatotoxicity in a timely manner.

This book is divided into two sections, comprising a total of six chapters. In the first section regarding drug-related hepatotoxicity, the introductory chapter briefly summarized the current controversy regarding glucocorticoids for acute severe drug-induced liver injury, chapter 2 reviewed various pharmacological therapies for drug-induced liver injury, chapter 3 discussed the role of gut microbiota in the management of drug-induced liver injury, and chapter 4 introduced the significance of dual-energy computed tomography for the evaluation of amiodarone-induced hepatotoxicity. In the second section, regarding hepatotoxicity in other aspects, chapter 5 reviewed the metabolic hepatic alterations and diseases under hypoxic conditions, and chapter 6 explored the hepatoprotective activity of proline derivatives.

We sincerely hope that the contents of this book will be helpful to physicians and scientists in gaining a deeper understanding of the current knowledge of hepatotoxicity. Herein, we would like to express our sincere appreciation to the authors for their contributions. We are also indebted to IntechOpen Publishing Process Manager Josip Knapic for his valuable assistance in preparing this book.

Dr. Xingshun Qi
Department of Gastroenterology,
General Hospital of Northern Theater Command,
Shenyang, China

Dr. Xiaofeng Liu
Department of Gastroenterology,
The 960th Hospital of Chinese PLA,
Jinan, China

Section 1

Drug-Related Hepatotoxicity

Chapter 1

Introductory Chapter: Glucocorticoids for Acute Severe Drug-Induced Liver Injury – Current Controversy

Xingshun Qi and Xiaofeng Liu

1. Introduction

Nowadays, drug-induced liver injury (DILI) is common in our daily clinical practice. It is likely that DILI can progress to acute liver failure or develop to chronic liver injury. It is important to prevent disease progression in acute DILI cases. Response to conventional drugs is unsatisfactory. It seems that glucocorticoids can achieve further clinical benefits in such cases.

2. Recommendations from guidelines and consensus

There is a controversy in the role of glucocorticoids for the treatment of DILI among practice guidelines and consensus. The European Association for the Study of the Liver (EASL) clinical practice guideline published in 2019 indicates that "routine use of corticosteroid treatment may not be substantiated in idiosyncratic DILI" [1]. Certainly, the EASL guideline also states that corticosteroid can be considered for DILI with hypersensitivity features. The Asia Pacific Association of the Study of Liver consensus guideline published in 2021 indicates that "N-Acetylcysteine combined with prednisolone improves liver biochemistries and function in flupirtine induced DILI" [2]. Meanwhile, the APASL consensus also recommends steroids for hepatoxicity from immune checkpoint inhibitors (ICIs) and biologics and drug-induced autoimmune-like hepatitis. The American Association for the Study of the Liver (AASLD) practice guidance published in 2022 indicates "corticosteriods given for 1-3 months may be beneficial in selected patients with idiosyncratic DILI, including those with hypersensitivity features, drug reaction with eosinophilia and systemic symptoms, and autoimmune features on liver biopsy" [3]. However, it also states that the optimal dose and duration of corticosteroids are unclear due to the absence of controlled clinical trials. The Chinese practice guideline published in 2023 suggested the absence of high-quality evidence regarding the use of corticosteroids as a routine treatment of DILI but recommended that it should be cautiously used for autoimmune-induced DILI with hypersensitivity and autoimmune-like characteristics and ICI-related hepatotoxicity [4]. Collectively, the recommendations from various guidelines were unclear, primarily because the current evidence regarding the use of glucocorticoids for the treatment of DILI remains greatly insufficient.

3. Evidence from studies

There are some scattered case reports regarding successful treatment of severe DILI by glucocorticoids [5, 6]. Additionally, there is also some low-quality evidence from retrospective studies regarding the use of glucocorticoids in severe DILI. In an early study conducted in the Peking University First Hospital, Hou et al. retrospectively analyzed the outcomes of 70 patients with hepatocellular DILI and total bilirubin level ≧ 10 upper limit of normal, of whom 20 were treated with steroids. The rate of disease resolution was significantly higher in patients who were treated with steroids than those who were not treated with steroids (100% versus 74%, P = 0.029) [7]. The mortality was also lower in patients who were treated with steroids than those who were not treated with steroids (0% versus 12%, P = 0.243), but the difference was not statistically significant. In another retrospective study performed in the Changzheng Hospital of the Second Military Medical University, Hu et al. separately evaluated the effects of corticosteroids in DILI patients with total bilirubin level of 85.5 umol/L and 243 umol/L [8]. In patients with a total bilirubin level of 85.5 umol/L, there was no significant difference in the average time from peak TBIL level to 50% reduction (12 ± 7 versus 14 ± 15 days, P = 0.303) or normal (50 ± 46 versus 49 ± 46 days, P = 0.918) and rate of death (9.4% versus 9.2%, P = 0.966) between steroids and no-steroids groups. In the patients with a total bilirubin level of 243 umol/L, the average time from peak TBIL level to 50% reduction was shorter in the steroids group than the no-steroids group (12 ± 6 versus 17 ± 12 days, P = 0.039), but there was no significant difference in the average time from peak TBIL level to normal between steroids and no-steroids groups (61 ± 56 versus 61 ± 37 days, P = 0.971). Additionally, there was no benefit of corticosteroids on decreasing the overall mortality. Wan et al. from the Second Affiliated Hospital of Kunming Medical University also conducted a retrospective observational study and found that prednisone was not beneficial for reduction of disease severity or improvement of overall survival in patients with severe DILI [9]. Besides, by retrospectively reviewing the data in 570 hospitalized Chinese patients with DILI, Pang et al. from the Peking University First Hospital did not demonstrate any significant benefit in the normalization of laboratory parameters [10].

4. Conclusions

Collectively, the role of glucocorticoids in management of DILI remains unclear. In future, high-quality studies, especially randomized controlled trials, are very necessary, as mentioned in a recent systematic review [11].

Author details

Xingshun Qi[1]* and Xiaofeng Liu[2]*

1 Department of Gastroenterology, General Hospital of Northern Theater Command, Shenyang, Liaoning Province, China

2 Department of Gastroenterology, The 960th Hospital of Chinese PLA, Jinan, Shandong Province, China

*Address all correspondence to: xingshunqi@126.com and liuxf0531@126.com

References

[1] EASL Clinical Practice Guidelines. Drug-induced liver injury. Journal of Hepatology. 2019;**70**(6):1222-1261

[2] Devarbhavi H, Aithal G, Treeprasertsuk S, Takikawa H, Mao Y, Shasthry SM, et al. Drug-induced liver injury: Asia Pacific Association of Study of liver consensus guidelines. Hepatology International. 2021;**15**(2):258-282

[3] Fontana RJ, Liou I, Reuben A, Suzuki A, Fiel MI, Lee W, et al. AASLD practice guidance on drug, herbal, and dietary supplement-induced liver injury. Hepatology. 2023;77(3):1036-1065

[4] Mao Y, Ma S, Liu C, Liu X, Su M, Li D, et al. Chinese guideline for the diagnosis and treatment of drug-induced liver injury: An update. Hepatology International. 2024;**18**(2):384-419

[5] Chai L, Wang R, Teschke R, Jin S, Deng J, Qi X. Successful corticosteroid therapy for severe liver injury secondary to herbal traditional Chinese medicine, mega defends X, assessed for causality by the updated RUCAM: A case report. Medicine (Baltimore). 2024;**103**(34):e39439

[6] Bai Z, Li H, Zheng K, Zhang J, Zhang X, Deng J, et al. A good response to glucocorticoid for sub-acute liver failure: A case report. Translational Gastroenterology and Hepatology. 2018;**3**:25

[7] Hou FQ, Zeng Z, Wang GQ. Hospital admissions for drug-induced liver injury: Clinical features, therapy, and outcomes. Cell Biochemistry and Biophysics. 2012;**64**(2):77-83

[8] Hu PF, Wang PQ, Chen H, Hu XF, Xie QP, Shi J, et al. Beneficial effect of corticosteroids for patients with severe drug-induced liver injury. Journal of Digestive Diseases. 2016;**17**(9):618-627

[9] Wan YM, Wu JF, Li YH, Wu HM, Wu XN, Xu Y. Prednisone is not beneficial for the treatment of severe drug-induced liver injury: An observational study (STROBE compliant). Medicine (Baltimore). 2019;**98**(26):e15886

[10] Pang L, Yang W, Hou F. Features and outcomes from a retrospective study of 570 hospitalized Chinese patients with drug-induced liver injury. Clinics and Research in Hepatology and Gastroenterology. 2018;**42**(1):48-56

[11] Björnsson ES, Vucic V, Stirnimann G, Robles-Díaz M. Role of corticosteroids in drug-induced liver injury. A systematic review. Frontiers in Pharmacology. 2022;**13**:820724

Chapter 2

Pharmacological Therapy for Drug-Induced Liver Injury

Qinke Wu, Ting Wang, Qianqian Li, Fei Gao, Chenghai Liu and Xingshun Qi

Abstract

Drug-induced liver injury (DILI) refers to a type of liver dysfunction induced by various drugs or their metabolites, which can be life-threatening. Its incidence is increasing gradually, and it has become a non-negligible global health burden. In daily life, many common medications can lead to DILI. However, there is still no single indicator which is specific for the diagnosis of DILI, and the medications for the treatment of DILI are clinically diverse. In addition, pharmacological therapy also faces additional challenges in some special populations with DILI, such as elderly people, children, and pregnant women. This chapter aims to summarize the current overview of various drugs to treat DILI in clinical practice.

Keywords: drug-induced liver injury (DILI), pharmacotherapy, hepatoprotective drug, acetaminophen (APAP), N-acetylcysteine (NAC), glycyrrhetinic acid preparation (GAP), antioxidants, silymarin, ursodeoxycholic acid (UDCA), L-carnitine (LC), tiopronin (TP), polyene phosphatidylcholine (PPC), S-adenosyl-methionine (SAMe), glucocorticoids (GCs)

1. Introduction

Drug-induced liver injury (DILI) refers to a type of liver injury induced by various drugs or their metabolites [1], which will prolong the duration of hospitalization, increase the cost, and decrease the quality of life for patients [2]. In Western countries, DILI has become the most common cause of acute liver failure (ALF) [3]. In Asian countries, its incidence is also gradually increasing, accounting for up to 4–10% of hospitalized patients [4, 5]. Currently, DILI has become a global burden of diseases that cannot be ignored [6]. Risk factors for DILI include advanced age, female gender, drug interactions, and drug hepatotoxicity [7–9]. Anticancer drugs, antibiotics, and nonsteroidal anti-inflammatory drugs are the leading causes of DILI [10–12]. In addition, traditional Chinese medicine and dietary supplements are major causes of DILI, but it is difficult to determine their potential toxicity due to their complex composition [13]. The proportion of traditional Chinese medicine-induced liver injury among all DILI cases is estimated as 25.71%, and it is gradually increased year by year [14]. Unfortunately, there is still no single indicator specific for DILI, which increases its diagnostic difficulty and uncertainty [15].

Nowadays, there are diverse drug treatment regimens [16]. In clinical practice, commonly used first-line medications for DILI include N-acetylcysteine (NAC), glycyrrhetinic acid preparation (GAP), ursodeoxycholic acid (UDCA), glucocorticoids (GCs), and glutathione (GSH). Specifically, GAP can effectively inhibit the release of inflammatory factors and reduce the inflammatory response of the liver; UDCA can improve the condition of cholestasis, promote the excretion of bile, and alleviate the toxicity of bile acids on hepatocytes; and GSH can maintain the intracellular redox balance and counteract the drug-induced oxidative stress damage [17–19]. Some other potentially effective drugs, such as cholestyramine (CSM) and clausenamide (CLA), are emerging.

At present, there are still many challenges in the pharmacological therapy for DILI. First, long-term follow-up and large-scale clinical studies regarding pharmacological therapy for DILI are scarce, so it may be risky. Second, there are differences in individual responses to medications, and some patients have poor efficacy and may experience adverse effects. In addition, drug-drug interactions add to the complexity of treatment. Thus, how to accurately select drugs, avoid adverse effects, and develop personalized treatment plans are still the current challenges to be overcome in the treatment of DILI. This chapter aims to summarize the current overview of various drugs to treat DILI in clinical practice.

2. Pathophysiology of DILI

The pathophysiology of DILI is multifaceted and complex. First, drugs or their metabolites can directly damage hepatocytes. For example, excessive acetaminophen (APAP) produces toxic N-acetyl-p-benzoquinone imine (NAPQI) [20]. Second, drugs may inhibit bile duct transporters, causing the accumulation of bile acids in the liver, which can lead to hepatocellular damage, liver fibrosis, and even cirrhosis [21]. Third, drugs activate the immune system by binding to hepatocyte proteins to form antigens, triggering the immune system to attack the hepatocytes, causing hepatocyte damage or necrosis [22]. Fourth, drugs disrupt mitochondrial function, causing metabolic disorders and oxidative stress, ultimately leading to hepatocyte swelling, degeneration, necrosis, and other lesions [23]. In addition, genetic polymorphisms (e.g., cytochrome P450 enzyme lineage) can affect drug metabolism and increase the risk of DILI [24]. Collectively, multiple factors are working together to cause DILI.

3. Pharmacological treatment for DILI

It is necessary to first discontinue the suspected medication related to DILI, and then intervene with the appropriate drugs [16]. Due to the complex pathophysiology of DILI, the efficacy of existing drugs remains limited. Based on the current evidence, the therapeutic drugs for DILI can be divided into four major categories: specific antidotes, non-specific hepatoprotective drugs, immunosuppressants, and potential drugs.

3.1 Specific antidotes

Currently, there are some specific antidotes for the treatment of DILI caused by certain drugs.

3.1.1 N-acetylcysteine

NAC is a sulfhydryl-containing GSH precursor compound with detoxifying, anti-inflammatory, and antioxidant effects [25]. It is the only antidote approved by the Food and Drug Administration for the treatment of APAP-induced endogenous DILI [26]. If an excessive amount of APAP was taken, the immediate use of NAC would effectively relieve symptoms, and the earlier it is taken, the better the effect will be [27].

NAC also seems to be effective for non-APAP-induced DILI. An open-label study suggests that NAC prevents anti-tuberculosis (TB) drug-induced DILI [28]. Lee et al. included 173 ALF patients who received NAC (n = 81) or placebo (n = 92) and demonstrated that patients who received NAC had a significantly higher transplant-free survival rate than those who received placebo (40% vs. 27%, P = 0.043) [29]. But Squires et al. failed to demonstrate that NAC improves survival in children with non-APAP ALF [30]. In conclusion, NAC is an antidote to APAP overdose-induced DILI and non-APAP-induced DILI, but not for children.

3.1.2 L-carnitine (LC)

LC, a class of amino acid analogs with anti-inflammatory and antioxidant properties, can be synthesized in small amounts by the human body, but mainly from daily intake of foods, such as red meat [31]. LC is a specific antidote for DILI caused by valproic acid (VPA). LC infusion may directly alleviate the LC deficiency induced by VPA and reduce hepatotoxicity. Meanwhile, Perrott et al. considered the use of LC in patients with acute VPA overdose and decreased consciousness based on the available evidence. Moreover, they recommended bolus intravenous infusion of LC at a dosage of 100 mg/kg, followed by 50 mg/kg every 8 hours with the maximum dosage not exceeding 3 g, until the ammonia level decreases, if initially elevated, and clinical symptoms are improved [32].

In addition, LC has been shown to be beneficial for preventing DILI caused by other drugs. A meta-analysis of 14 randomized controlled trials (RCTs) evaluated the efficacy of LC for various chronic liver diseases, and found that LC supplementation significantly reduced alanine aminotransferase (ALT) and aspartate aminotransferase (AST) levels in patients with chronic liver diseases [33]. Besides, Hatamkhani et al. demonstrated that anti-TB drugs combined with oral LC solution at a dosage of 2000 mg daily for 4 weeks significantly reduced the incidence of anti-TB drug-induced hepatotoxicity (ATDH) [34]. Taken together, LC, an antidote for VPA-induced DILI, has potential prophylactic effects on non-VPA-induced DILI.

3.2 Non-specific hepatoprotective drugs

Hepatoprotective drugs refer to a kind of drugs that prevent or reduce liver injury, promote liver cell regeneration, and thus improve liver function. Thus, various hepatoprotective drugs play an important role in the treatment of DILI.

3.2.1 Glycyrrhizic acid preparation

GAP, such as magnesium isoglycyrrhizate (MgIG) and compound glycyrrhizic acid, which is an extract preparation of *Glycyrrhiza glabra*, is widely used for the treatment of liver diseases [35]. GAP not only inhibits the release of multiple inflammatory mediators but also protects hepatocytes by reducing oxidative stress [36]. In 2015, MgIG was approved by the China Food and Drug Administration for the treatment of acute DILI [26]. A phase II clinical trial demonstrated that both low-dose MgIG and high-dose MgIG reduced ALT levels more significantly than thiopronin (TP) [37]. Besides, Yao et al. showed that GAP injection can effectively reduce ALT and AST levels in DILI patients with good safety [38]. Until now, GAP has been widely used in various countries to treat DILI [39]. In future, large-scale prospective studies are still needed to further explore the efficacy of GAP in DILI.

3.2.2 Silymarin

Silymarin is a flavonoid extracted from the seeds of the milk thistle [40]. It is a potent antioxidant, which can protect the structural integrity of hepatocytes and ensure the normal metabolic function of the liver [41]. Therefore, silymarin is more applicable for the hepatocyte injury type DILI. However, an RCT in Iran showed that folic acid significantly reduced ALT ($P = 0.04$) and AST ($P = 0.007$) levels in children with epileptic drug-induced DILI compared to silymarin [42]. Another RCT by Marjani et al. showed that silymarin had poor therapeutic effects on anti-TB drug-induced DILI [43]. Additionally, a meta-analysis evaluated the efficacy of several hepatoprotective drugs in decreasing AST and total bilirubin (TBIL) levels, and found that silymarin had lower efficacy [44]. On the other hand, silymarin, a natural plant extract, is safe with almost no adverse reactions and good tolerance [45, 46]. In conclusion, silymarin offers a safe option for the treatment of DILI, but its therapeutic efficacy is controversial.

3.2.3 Ursodeoxycholic acid

UDCA was originally extracted from bear bile, and can be artificially synthesized now [47]. UDCA can promote the secretion of bile acids and excretion of toxic metabolites, thus reducing the burden on the liver [18]. Accordingly, UDCA has long been used clinically for cholestatic DILI. Lang et al. showed that oral UDCA reversed the hepatotoxicity of ATDH [48]. Another study found that UDCA was effective and well-tolerated in children with anticonvulsant-induced hypertransaminasemia ($n = 22$) [49]. Moreover, UDCA also shows some preventive effects. A retrospective study by Kojima et al. suggested the prophylactic effect of UDCA against flutamide-induced hepatopathy in patients with prostate cancer [50]. A prospective study showed that UDCA prevents the hepatotoxicity of chemotherapy drugs in pediatric patients with B-cell acute lymphoblastic leukemia [51]. Based on the available evidence, UDCA should be beneficial for both the prevention and treatment of DILI, and is particularly indicated for cholestatic DILI.

3.2.4 Bicyclol

In 2004, bicyclol was approved in China as an anti-inflammatory and hepatoprotective drug for the treatment of various forms of liver injury [52]. Bicyclol can alleviate liver inflammation, enhance antioxidant capacity of hepatocytes, and promote hepatocyte repair and regeneration [53]. It can play an important role in the treatment of DILI presenting with a significantly elevated ALT, because it can rapidly reduce ALT levels and be favorable for hepatic recovery. In 2014, Wu et al. randomized patients with statin-induced liver injury into a treatment group (bicyclol 25 mg three times per day, n = 79) and a control group (polyene phosphatidylcholine [PPC] 456 mg three times per day, n = 78). After 4 weeks, the rate of ALT normalization was significantly higher in the treatment group than the control group (74.68% vs. 46.15%). Therefore, bisacodyl is safe and effective in the treatment of statin-induced DILI [54]. Meanwhile, Li et al. showed that oral administration of bicyclol at a dosage of 75 mg daily significantly reduced the incidence and extent of chemotherapeutic agent-induced liver damage in elderly patients with cancer [55]. In addition, a phase II trial in 2022 showed that bicyclol had better efficacy for the treatment of idiopathic acute DILI when it was taken three times a day at a dosage of 50 mg [56]. On the other hand, Chen et al. evaluated the pharmacoeconomics of bicyclol, diammonium glycyrrhizinate, and silibinin for the treatment of ATDH, and concluded that bicyclol was the most cost-effective therapy and the first choice for the treatment of ATDH [57]. In brief, bicyclol has excellent efficacy, safety, and affordability, making it one of the preferred drugs for the treatment of DILI.

3.2.5 Polyene phosphatidylcholine

PPC is purified from phospholipids extracted from soybeans, which can bind with the liver cell membrane to protect and repair hepatocytes [58]. Currently, PPC is widely used globally for the treatment of various liver diseases and is mainly used in China for the treatment of DILI. A retrospective study from China showed that both PPC and MgIG had positive efficacy in the treatment of DILI, resulting in a significant reduction in ALT levels, and that the safety and efficacy of these two drugs in treating DILI were comparable [59]. Notably, it should be used with caution in patients with bean allergies, primarily considering the ingredient of PPC. In conclusion, PPC is mainly used in China for the treatment of DILI, especially for DILI presenting with a significantly elevated ALT.

3.2.6 Tiopronin

TP, a sulfhydryl-containing glycine, can be detoxified by formulating non-toxic mixtures with toxic substances [60]. Li et al. included 150 patients with advanced colorectal cancer to assess the efficacy of TP infusion on chemotherapy-induced hepatotoxicity. Compared to the control group, the TP group had significantly lower proportions of abnormal mean ALT, AST, TBIL, and albumin levels. Therefore, TP reduced the incidence of chemotherapy-induced hepatotoxicity and enhanced the patients' tolerance to chemotherapy [61]. Wang et al. investigated the efficacy of MgIG on DILI, and showed a positive effect of TP [37]. In addition, a case report suggests that TP is effective for liver injury caused by long-term use of antiepileptic drugs, but more clinical studies are needed to determine the exact mechanism of action [62]. Collectively, TP is beneficial for the treatment of DILI, especially in patients who received chemotherapy.

3.2.7 S-adenosyl-methionine (SAMe)

SAMe is involved in numerous biochemical reactions in vivo as a methyl donor and precursor of physiological sulfhydryl compounds and has been referred to as a control switch for regulating liver function [63, 64]. Because the metabolism of exogenous SAMe is hardly affected by chronic liver diseases, it should be potentially more effective in the setting of chronic liver diseases [65]. Santini et al. administered SAMe supplementation orally to cancer patients (n = 50) who have anticancer chemotherapy-induced hepatotoxicity, and showed that SAMe could significantly reduce AST and ALT levels [66]. In addition, it has been shown to regulate the process of bile acid metabolism, relieve symptoms associated with cholestasis, and can be used during pregnancy [67, 68]. It has been confirmed that SAMe improves hepatic biochemical parameters and cholestatic symptoms [69]. It should be noted that SAMe is unstable in nature and requires attention to storage conditions and the time frame for use after configuration [70]. Collectively, SAMe can improve liver function in cholestatic DILI.

3.3 Immunosuppressants

Immunosuppressants play a key role in the treatment of DILI, especially immune-mediated injury. When certain drugs are administered to the human body, immune response is abnormally activated, triggering a series of inflammatory chain reactions [71]. Immunosuppressants inhibit the activation and proliferation of T-lymphocytes, thereby reducing the intensity of the attack on hepatocytes [72]. However, they are not omnipotent, and their use requires a rigorous assessment of the patient's condition, immune status, and potential risks.

GCs are steroid hormones secreted by the adrenal cortex. In clinical practice, empirical administration of GCs can effectively improve liver function in severe DILI [73, 74]. Wang et al. demonstrated that GC plus glycyrrhizin for chronic DILI can achieve both biochemical response and histological improvements with good safety [75]. A retrospective study strongly recommended short-term use of GCs in severe DILI patients with hyperbilirubinemia, which may improve liver injury and patient survival [76]. But another study demonstrated that GCs do not improve the cure rate of severe DILI, but can rapidly reduce TBIL at early stage [77]. A study from Iceland noted that GCs were effective for the treatment of infliximab-induced DILI, with normalization of liver function indices and no recurrence after long-term follow-up period [78]. However, it has also been shown that GCs are not beneficial for the treatment of DILI, and even harmful at a daily dosage of >40 mg [37]. In conclusion, GCs are effective for the treatment of DILI, but may trigger adverse effects, such as Cushing's syndrome. Therefore, clinicians need to accurately grasp the dosage and duration of GCs according to the patient's specific condition, and weigh the pros and cons of GCs before their use.

3.4 Potential drugs

Development of new potential agents has opened new avenues to strengthen the treatment efficacy. Notably, clinical studies of these agents are limited. Their potential benefits for treating DILI have been demonstrated in animal studies or in some cases, providing new options for the treatment of DILI in the future.

3.4.1 Cholestyramine

CSM, an anion-exchange resin, is not absorbed by the gastrointestinal tract after oral administration, and is excreted in the feces by irreversibly binding to bile acids in the intestinal tract, forming an insoluble complex [79]. Thus, CSM reduces the hepatic-intestinal circulation of bile acids and lowers the concentration of bile acids in the bile, which in turn attenuates the toxic effects of bile acids on hepatocytes. According to the European Association for the Study of the Liver guidelines, the use of CSM is recommended for ALF induced by leflunomide to accelerate drug clearance [80]. In two cases of DILI where UDCA and GCs were ineffective, oral CSM immediately relieved jaundice and pruritus [81]. Besides, terbinafine has been reported to potentially cause cholestatic DILI [82]. The Asia Pacific Association for the Study of the Liver guidelines recommend oral CSM for terbinafine-induced DILI. In conclusion, CSM is indicated for cholestatic DILI and alleviation of itchy skin.

3.4.2 Glutathione

GSH is one of the most important antioxidants in cells, and intracellular GSH levels are crucial for maintaining redox homeostasis [19]. When NAC binds toxic NAPQI, it reduces the body's natural storage of GSH, leading to hepatocyte necrosis. Many drugs used to treat DILI, such as NAC, SAMe, MgIG, and UDCA, work by increasing the GSH level in the body [83]. They are GSH precursors, and can promote GSH production. Similarly, DILI can be treated with direct GSH supplementation. If GSH is decreased in vivo, it indicates a greater susceptibility to oxidative stress, thus GSH has potential as a biochemical indicator of DILI [84]. Currently, experimental researches focus on the molecular signaling pathway of GSH action, and more clinical studies are needed to provide theoretical support for its role in the treatment of DILI.

3.4.3 Clausenamide

CLA is an amide compound isolated from the leaves of the plant *Clausena lansium* [85]. It is able to regulate many key cellular signaling pathways in the liver, weakening the attack of a large amount of reactive oxygen clusters on hepatocytes, and maintaining normal cellular redox homeostasis [86]. Wu et al. showed that CLA is an active initiator for generating GSH in the liver [87]. In addition, ferroptosis is a widely discussed topic related to DILI. Wang et al. proposed the role of CLA for the treatment of APAP-induced DILI by inhibiting hepatocyte ferroptosis [88]. Collectively, CLA should be promising for the treatment of DILI.

4. Pharmacological therapy for special populations with DILI (SP-DILI)

When DILI develop in SP-DILI groups, such as elderly people, children, and pregnant women, additional challenges are faced. Therefore, we need to pay great attention to the treatment of DILI in SP-DILI and deeply explore the efficacy and safety of medications.

4.1 Elderly people

Elderly people (65 years and over) have an increased incidence of various diseases, require multiple medications to maintain their health, and are more susceptible to DILI than the general population. Weersink et al. found increased rates of comorbidities and polypharmacy and more severe DILI with increasing age in all elderly groups [89]. When medications were administrated to elderly patients with DILI, there is a need for consideration regarding decreased ability to metabolize medications in the elderly. Moreover, there is a gradual shift in the pattern of liver injury toward cholestasis in the elderly, so the drugs indicated for cholestatic DILI are favored [7]. Collectively, elderly patients with DILI need a comprehensive selection of therapeutic agents according to the age, comorbidities, and type of liver injury. Future studies involving more elderly patients with DILI are needed.

4.2 Children

In children, the liver is still under development, and the drug metabolism enzyme system is incomplete [90]. In the United States, the leading causes of DILI in children are antimicrobials (51%) and antiepileptic drugs (21%), especially minocycline and valproate [91]. Physicians should be aware of their potential risk of liver damage in children. And the choice of medications must be made carefully in children with DILI. On the one hand, the choice of dosage form is crucial, and the preference should be given to oral liquid formulations that are easily accepted by children and also allow for more precise control of dosage [92]. On the other hand, given the sensitivity of children to drug reactions, the dosage should be calculated accurately according to the age and weight throughout the treatment. At the same time, we should be aware of the potential effects of drugs on the children's growth and development and fully weigh whether they interfere with the absorption and metabolism of nutrients.

4.3 Pregnant women

In pregnant women, DILI is complex and can adversely affect both mother and fetus. When choosing medications for DILI, we must not only consider their efficacy, but also avoid the use of teratogenic drugs. Second, it is important to regularly examine the fetus and the mother's liver function. In addition, multidisciplinary collaboration plays an integral role in the treatment of DILI. Obstetricians focus on the safety of mother and fetus, while hepatologists focus on the efficacy of pharmacological therapy for DILI. In the future, it is necessary to summarize adverse events during pregnancy and provide more evidence on the safety of medication for pregnant women with DILI.

5. Conclusion

Currently, DILI is a challenge in the global medical field. Specific antidotes (NAC and LC) are well-targeted but have limited application, hepatoprotective drugs (GAP, silymarin, and UDCA, etc.) are beneficial but lack high-quality clinical studies, immunosuppressants (GCs) are rapidly effective but potentially risky, and potential drugs (CSM, GSH, and CLA) require further assessment. Moreover, it is important to pay attention to the pharmacological treatment of DILI in SP-DILI.

Authors' contributions

Qinke Wu reviewed and searched the literature and wrote the first draft.

Ting Wang, Qianqian Li, Fei Gao, and Chenghai Liu discussed the findings, revised the manuscript, and gave critical comments.

Xingshun Qi conceived and supervised the work, reviewed and searched the literature, and revised the manuscript.

All authors participated in the discussion of this study protocol, gave critical comments on this manuscript, and approved this submission.

Funding

Liaoning Provincial Science and Technology Plan Joint Plan (Technology Research and Attack Plan Project) 2024JH2/102600285.

Conflict of interest

None.

Author details

Qinke Wu[1,2†], Ting Wang[1,2†], Qianqian Li[1†], Fei Gao[1†], Chenghai Liu[3*] and Xingshun Qi[1,2*]

1 Department of Gastroenterology, General Hospital of Northern Theater Command (Teaching Hospital of Shenyang Pharmaceutical University), Shenyang, China

2 Department of Clinical Pharmacy, Shenyang Pharmaceutical University, Shenyang, China

3 Shuguang Hospital, Shanghai University of Traditional Chinese Medicine, Shanghai, China

*Address all correspondence to: chenghai.liu@outlook.com and xingshunqi@126.com

† These authors contributed equally to this work.

References

[1] Bjornsson HK, Bjornsson ES. Drug-induced liver injury: Pathogenesis, epidemiology, clinical features, and practical management. European Journal of Internal Medicine. 2022;**97**(6):26-31

[2] Licata A. Adverse drug reactions and organ damage: The liver. European Journal of Internal Medicine. 2016;**28**(8):9-16

[3] Reuben A, Koch DG, Lee WM, Acute Liver Failure Study Group. Drug-induced acute liver failure: Results of a U.S. multicenter, prospective study. Hepatology. 2010;**52**(6):2065-2076

[4] Sobhonslidsuk A, Poovorawan K, Soonthornworasiri N, Pan-Ngum W, Phaosawasdi K. The incidence, presentation, outcomes, risk of mortality and economic data of drug-induced liver injury from a national database in Thailand: A population-base study. BMC Gastroenterology. 2016;**16**(1):135

[5] Suk KT, Kim DJ, Kim CH, et al. A prospective nationwide study of drug-induced liver injury in Korea. The American Journal of Gastroenterology. 2012;**107**(9):1380-1387

[6] Li M, Wang Y, Lv TT, et al. Mapping the incidence of drug-induced liver injury: A systematic review and meta-analysis. Journal of Digestive Diseases. 2023;**24**(5):332-339

[7] Lucena MI, Sanabria J, Garcia-Cortes M, Stephens C, Andrade RJ. Drug-induced liver injury in older people. The Lancet Gastroenterology & Hepatology. 2020;**5**(9):862-874

[8] Floreani A, Bizzaro D, Shalaby S, Taliani G, Burra P, Special Interest Group Gender in Hepatology of the Italian Association for the Study of the Liver. Sex disparity and drug-induced liver injury. Digestive and Liver Disease. 2023;**55**(1):21-28

[9] Todorovic Vukotic N, Dordevic J, Pejic S, Dordevic N, Pajovic SB. Antidepressants- and antipsychotics-induced hepatotoxicity. Archives of Toxicology. 2021;**95**(3):767-789

[10] Pocurull A, Moreta MJ, Heitman D, et al. Anticancer drugs are the first cause of drug-induced liver injury in a reference hospital. Liver International. 2024;**44**(2):286-292

[11] Bjornsson ES. Drug-induced liver injury due to antibiotics. Scandinavian Journal of Gastroenterology. 2017;**52**(6-7):617-623

[12] Bessone F. Non-steroidal anti-inflammatory drugs: What is the actual risk of liver damage? World Journal of Gastroenterology. 2010;**16**(45):5651-5661

[13] de Boer YS, Sherker AH. Herbal and dietary supplement-induced liver injury. Clinics in Liver Disease. 2017;**21**(1):135-149

[14] Wang R, Qi X, Yoshida EM, et al. Clinical characteristics and outcomes of traditional Chinese medicine-induced liver injury: A systematic review. Expert Review of Gastroenterology & Hepatology. 2018;**12**(4):425-434

[15] Andrade RJ, Robles-Diaz M. Diagnostic and prognostic assessment of suspected drug-induced liver injury in clinical practice. Liver International. 2020;**40**(1):6-17

[16] Hassan A, Fontana RJ. The diagnosis and management of idiosyncratic

drug-induced liver injury. Liver International. 2019;**39**(1):31-41

[17] Wang CY, Kao TC, Lo WH, Yen GC. Glycyrrhizic acid and 18beta-glycyrrhetinic acid modulate lipopolysaccharide-induced inflammatory response by suppression of NF-kappaB through PI3K p110delta and p110gamma inhibitions. Journal of Agricultural and Food Chemistry. 2011;**59**(14):7726-7733

[18] Paumgartner G, Beuers U. Mechanisms of action and therapeutic efficacy of ursodeoxycholic acid in cholestatic liver disease. Clinics in Liver Disease. 2004;**8**(1):67-81

[19] Forman HJ, Zhang H, Rinna A. Glutathione: Overview of its protective roles, measurement, and biosynthesis. Molecular Aspects of Medicine. 2009;**30**(1-2):1-12

[20] Cai X, Cai H, Wang J, et al. Molecular pathogenesis of acetaminophen-induced liver injury and its treatment options. Journal of Zhejiang University. Science. B. 2022;**23**(4):265-285

[21] Bhamidimarri KR, Schiff E. Drug-induced cholestasis. Clinics in Liver Disease. 2013;**17**(4):519-531

[22] Yan M, Huo Y, Yin S, Hu H. Mechanisms of acetaminophen-induced liver injury and its implications for therapeutic interventions. Redox Biology. 2018;**17**(10):274-283

[23] Kuretu A, Arineitwe C, Mothibe M, Ngubane P, Khathi A, Sibiya N. Drug-induced mitochondrial toxicity: Risks of developing glucose handling impairments. Frontiers in Endocrinology (Lausanne). 2023;**14**:1123928

[24] Andrade RJ, Robles M, Ulzurrun E, Lucena MI. Drug-induced liver injury: Insights from genetic studies. Pharmacogenomics. 2009;**10**(9):1467-1487

[25] Dekhuijzen PN. Antioxidant properties of N-acetylcysteine: Their relevance in relation to chronic obstructive pulmonary disease. The European Respiratory Journal. 2004;**23**(4):629-636

[26] Li M, Luo Q, Tao Y, Sun X, Liu C. Pharmacotherapies for drug-induced liver injury: A current literature review. Frontiers in Pharmacology. 2021;**12**:806249

[27] Williamson K, Wahl MS, Mycyk MB. Direct comparison of 20-hour IV, 36-hour oral, and 72-hour oral acetylcysteine for treatment of acute acetaminophen poisoning. American Journal of Therapeutics. 2013;**20**(1):37-40

[28] Baniasadi S, Eftekhari P, Tabarsi P, et al. Protective effect of N-acetylcysteine on antituberculosis drug-induced hepatotoxicity. European Journal of Gastroenterology & Hepatology. 2010;**22**(10):1235-1238

[29] Lee WM, Hynan LS, Rossaro L, et al. Intravenous N-acetylcysteine improves transplant-free survival in early stage non-acetaminophen acute liver failure. Gastroenterology. 2009;**137**(3):856-864, 864.e851

[30] Squires RH, Dhawan A, Alonso E, et al. Intravenous N-acetylcysteine in pediatric patients with nonacetaminophen acute liver failure: A placebo-controlled clinical trial. Hepatology. 2013;**57**(4):1542-1549

[31] Pekala J, Patkowska-Sokola B, Bodkowski R, et al. L-carnitine—Metabolic functions and meaning in humans life. Current Drug Metabolism. 2011;**12**(7):667-678

[32] Perrott J, Murphy NG, Zed PJ. L-carnitine for acute valproic acid overdose: A systematic review of published cases. The Annals of Pharmacotherapy. 2010;**44**(7-8):1287-1293

[33] Oh H, Park CH, Jun DW. Impact of l-carnitine supplementation on liver enzyme normalization in patients with chronic liver disease: A meta-analysis of randomized trials. Journal of Personalized Medicine. 2022;**12**(7):1053

[34] Hatamkhani S, Khalili H, Karimzadeh I, Dashti-Khavidaki S, Abdollahi A, Jafari S. Carnitine for prevention of antituberculosis drug-induced hepatotoxicity: A randomized, clinical trial. Journal of Gastroenterology and Hepatology. 2014;**29**(5):997-1004

[35] Li X, Sun R, Liu R. Natural products in licorice for the therapy of liver diseases: Progress and future opportunities. Pharmacological Research. 2019;**144**(17):210-226

[36] Abo El-Magd NF, El-Mesery M, El-Karef A, El-Shishtawy MM. Glycyrrhizin ameliorates high fat diet-induced obesity in rats by activating NrF2 pathway. Life Sciences. 2018;**193**(12):159-170

[37] Wang Y, Wang Z, Gao M, et al. Efficacy and safety of magnesium isoglycyrrhizinate injection in patients with acute drug-induced liver injury: A phase II trial. Liver International. 2019;**39**(11):2102-2111

[38] Yao L, Zhang J, Jin J, et al. An analysis of the efficacy and safety of compound glycyrrhizin injections in the treatment of drug-induced liver injury using a nationwide database. International Journal of Clinical Pharmacy. 2022;**44**(3):731-740

[39] Tian X, Gan W, Nie Y, et al. Clinical efficacy and security of glycyrrhizic acid preparation in the treatment of anti-SARS-CoV-2 drug-induced liver injury: A protocol of systematic review and meta-analysis. BMJ Open. 2021;**11**(7):e051484

[40] Abenavoli L, Capasso R, Milic N, Capasso F. Milk thistle in liver diseases: Past, present, future. Phytotherapy Research. 2010;**24**(10):1423-1432

[41] Surai PF. Silymarin as a natural antioxidant: An overview of the current evidence and perspectives. Antioxidants (Basel). 2015;**4**(1):204-247

[42] Asgarshirazi M, Shariat M, Sheikh M. Comparison of efficacy of folic acid and silymarin in the management of antiepileptic drug induced liver injury: A randomized clinical trial. Hepatobiliary & Pancreatic Diseases International. 2017;**16**(3):296-302

[43] Marjani M, Fahim F, Sadr M, et al. Evaluation of Silymarin for management of anti-tuberculosis drug induced liver injury: A randomized clinical trial. Gastroenterology and Hepatology from Bed to Bench. 2019;**12**(2):138-142

[44] Li C, Yang X, Quan Y, Wu A, Wang Y. Network meta-analysis of different liver protective drugs in the treatment of drug-induced liver injury. Medicine (Baltimore). 2023;**102**(50):e36538

[45] Abenavoli L, Izzo AA, Milic N, Cicala C, Santini A, Capasso R. Milk thistle (*Silybum marianum*): A concise overview on its chemistry, pharmacological, and nutraceutical uses in liver diseases. Phytotherapy Research. 2018;**32**(11):2202-2213

[46] Soleimani V, Delghandi PS, Moallem SA, Karimi G. Safety and toxicity of silymarin, the major

constituent of milk thistle extract: An updated review. Phytotherapy Research. 2019;**33**(6):1627-1638

[47] Song P, Zhang X, Feng W, et al. Biological synthesis of ursodeoxycholic acid. Frontiers in Microbiology. 2023;**14**:1140662

[48] Lang SM, Ortmann J, Rostig S, Schiffl H. Ursodeoxycholic acid attenuates hepatotoxicity of multidrug treatment of mycobacterial infections: A prospective pilot study. International Journal of Mycobacteriology. 2019;**8**(1):89-92

[49] Asgarshirazi M, Shariat M, Dalili H, Keihanidoost Z. Ursodeoxycholic acid can improve liver transaminase quantities in children with anticonvulsant drugs hepatotoxicity: A pilot study. Acta Medica Iranica. 2015;**53**(6):351-355

[50] Kojima M, Kamoi K, Ukimura O, et al. Clinical utility of ursodeoxycholic acid in preventing flutamide-induced hepatopathy in patients with prostate cancer: A preliminary study. International Journal of Urology. 2002;**9**(1):42-46

[51] Mohammed Saif M, Farid SF, Khaleel SA, Sabry NA, El-Sayed MH. Hepatoprotective efficacy of ursodeoxycholic acid in pediatrics acute lymphoblastic leukemia. Pediatric Hematology and Oncology. 2012;**29**(7):627-632

[52] Zhao T, Mao L, Yu Z, et al. Therapeutic potential of bicyclol in liver diseases: Lessons from a synthetic drug based on herbal derivative in traditional Chinese medicine. International Immunopharmacology. 2021;**91**:107308

[53] Liu GT, Li Y, Wei HL, Zhang H, Xu JY, Yu LH. Mechanism of protective action of bicyclol against CCl-induced liver injury in mice. Liver International. 2005;**25**(4):872-879

[54] Naiqiong W, Liansheng W, Zhanying H, et al. A multicenter and randomized controlled trial of bicyclol in the treatment of statin-induced liver injury. Medical Science Monitor. 2017;**23**(7):5760-5766

[55] Li X, Zhou J, Chen S, et al. Role of bicyclol in preventing chemotherapeutic agent-induced liver injury in patients over 60 years of age with cancer. The Journal of International Medical Research. 2014;**42**(4):906-914

[56] Du Y, Gu J, Yang Y, et al. Efficacy and safety of bicyclol for treating patients with antituberculosis drug-induced liver injury. The International Journal of Tuberculosis and Lung Disease. 2024;**28**(1):6-12

[57] Chen Y, Ye P, Ren C, et al. Pharmacoeconomics of three therapeutic schemes for anti-tuberculosis therapy induced liver injury in China. Open Medicine (Warsaw, Poland). 2018;**13**(11):53-63

[58] Mak KM, Shekhar AC. Soybean polyenylphosphatidylcholine (PPC) is beneficial in liver and extrahepatic tissue injury: An update in experimental research. The Anatomical Record (Hoboken). 2024;**307**(6):2162-2186

[59] Lei X, Zhang J, Xu Q, et al. Exploring the efficacy and safety of polyene phosphatidylcholine for treatment of drug-induced liver injury using the Roussel Uclaf causality assessment method: A propensity score matching comparison. The Journal of International Medical Research. 2021;**49**(8):3000605211039810

[60] Kumar A, Estes Bright LM, Garren MRS, Manuel J, Shome A,

Handa H. Chemical modification of tiopronin for dual management of cystinuria and associated bacterial infections. ACS Applied Materials & Interfaces. 2023;**15**(37):43332-43344

[61] Li XP, Wen F, Yang W, et al. The role of tiopronin for the prevention of chemotherapy-related liver toxicity in advanced colorectal cancer patients treated with mFOLFOX7: A prospective analysis. Tumori. 2014;**100**(4):446-451

[62] Rose GA. Tiopronin in epilepsy. Lancet. 1986;**1**(8478):452

[63] Chiang PK, Gordon RK, Tal J, et al. S-Adenosylmethionine and methylation. The FASEB Journal. 1996;**10**(4):471-480

[64] Mato JM, Corrales FJ, Lu SC, Avila MA. S-Adenosylmethionine: A control switch that regulates liver function. The FASEB Journal. 2002;**16**(1):15-26

[65] Kaye GL, Blake JC, Burroughs AK. Metabolism of exogenous S-adenosyl-L-methionine in patients with liver disease. Drugs. 1990;**40 Suppl 3**(5):124-128

[66] Santini D, Vincenzi B, Massacesi C, et al. S-adenosylmethionine (AdoMet) supplementation for treatment of chemotherapy-induced liver injury. Anticancer Research. 2003;**23**(6D):5173-5179

[67] Frezza M, Surrenti C, Manzillo G, Fiaccadori F, Bortolini M, Di Padova C. Oral S-adenosylmethionine in the symptomatic treatment of intrahepatic cholestasis. A double-blind, placebo-controlled study. Gastroenterology. 1990;**99**(1):211-215

[68] Lu SC, Mato JM. S-adenosylmethionine in liver health, injury, and cancer. Physiological Reviews. 2012;**92**(4):1515-1542

[69] Noureddin M, Sander-Struckmeier S, Mato JM. Early treatment efficacy of S-adenosylmethionine in patients with intrahepatic cholestasis: A systematic review. World Journal of Hepatology. 2020;**12**(2):46-63

[70] Hoffman JL. Chromatographic analysis of the chiral and covalent instability of S-adenosyl-L-methionine. Biochemistry. 1986;**25**(15):4444-4449

[71] Liu W, Zeng X, Liu Y, et al. The immunological mechanisms and immune-based biomarkers of drug-induced liver injury. Frontiers in Pharmacology. 2021;**12**:723940

[72] Nayak SP, Bagchi B, Roy S. Effects of immunosuppressants on T-cell dynamics: Understanding from a generic coarse-grained immune network model. Journal of Biosciences. 2022;**47**(4):70

[73] Hou FQ, Zeng Z, Wang GQ. Hospital admissions for drug-induced liver injury: Clinical features, therapy, and outcomes. Cell Biochemistry and Biophysics. 2012;**64**(2):77-83

[74] Niu H, Ma J, Medina-Caliz I, et al. Potential benefit and lack of serious risk from corticosteroids in drug-induced liver injury: An international, multicentre, propensity score-matched analysis. Alimentary Pharmacology & Therapeutics. 2023;**57**(8):886-896

[75] Wang JB, Huang A, Wang Y, et al. Corticosteroid plus glycyrrhizin therapy for chronic drug- or herb-induced liver injury achieves biochemical and histological improvements: A randomised open-label trial. Alimentary Pharmacology & Therapeutics. 2022;**55**(10):1297-1310

[76] Hu PF, Wang PQ, Chen H, et al. Beneficial effect of corticosteroids for

patients with severe drug-induced liver injury. Journal of Digestive Diseases. 2016;**17**(9):618-627

[77] Wu H, Yan W, Liu K, Jing J, Ye W. Propensity score matching-based analysis of the effect of corticosteroids in treating severe drug-induced liver injury. Clinics and Research in Hepatology and Gastroenterology. 2024;**48**(9):102472

[78] Bjornsson HK, Gudbjornsson B, Bjornsson ES. Infliximab-induced liver injury: Clinical phenotypes, autoimmunity and the role of corticosteroid treatment. Journal of Hepatology. 2022;**76**(1):86-92

[79] Thompson WG. Cholestyramine. Canadian Medical Association Journal. 1971;**104**(4):305-309

[80] European Association for the Study of the Liver. EASL Clinical Practice Guidelines: Drug-induced liver injury. Journal of Hepatology. 2019;**70**(6):1222-1261

[81] Tani M, Hayashi Y, Okamoto S, et al. Rapid improvement of icterus and pruritus by the oral administration of colestimide in two cases of drug-induced hepatitis. Internal Medicine. 2001;**40**(11):1098-1103

[82] Mallat A, Zafrani ES, Metreau JM, Dhumeaux D. Terbinafine-induced prolonged cholestasis with reduction of interlobular bile ducts. Digestive Diseases and Sciences. 1997;**42**(7):1486-1488

[83] Zeng L, Jin X, Xiao QA, et al. Ferroptosis: Action and mechanism of chemical/drug-induced liver injury. Drug and Chemical Toxicology. 2024;**47**(6):1300-1311

[84] Liu K, Kang B, Luo X, et al. Redox-activated contrast-enhanced T(1)-weighted imaging visualizes glutathione-mediated biotransformation dynamics in the liver. ACS Nano. 2021;**15**(11):17831-17841

[85] Huang X, Wang M, Zhong S, Xu B. Comprehensive review of phytochemical profiles and health-promoting effects of different portions of Wampee (*Clausena lansium*). ACS Omega. 2023;**8**(30):26699-26714

[86] Xu MZ, Lee WS, Han JM, et al. Antioxidant and anti-inflammatory activities of N-acetyldopamine dimers from Periostracum Cicadae. Bioorganic & Medicinal Chemistry. 2006;**14**(23):7826-7834

[87] Wu YQ, Liu LD, Wei HL, Liu GT. Different effects of nine clausenamide ennatiomers on liver glutathione biosynthesis and glutathione S-transferase activity in mice. Acta Pharmacologica Sinica. 2006;**27**(8):1024-1028

[88] Wang M, Liu CY, Wang T, et al. (+)-Clausenamide protects against drug-induced liver injury by inhibiting hepatocyte ferroptosis. Cell Death & Disease. 2020;**11**(9):781

[89] Weersink RA, Alvarez-Alvarez I, Medina-Caliz I, et al. Clinical characteristics and outcome of drug-induced liver injury in the older patients: From the young-old to the oldest-old. Clinical Pharmacology and Therapeutics. 2021;**109**(4):1147-1158

[90] Kearns GL, Abdel-Rahman SM, Alander SW, Blowey DL, Leeder JS, Kauffman RE. Developmental pharmacology—Drug disposition, action, and therapy in infants and children. The New England Journal of Medicine. 2003;**349**(12):1157-1167

[91] Monge-Urrea F, Montijo-Barrios E. Drug-induced liver injury in pediatrics.

Journal of Pediatric Gastroenterology and Nutrition. 2022;**75**(4):391-395

[92] Kamphuis AEM, Bamford A, Tagarro A, et al. Optimising paediatric HIV treatment: Recent developments and future directions. Paediatric Drugs. 2024;**26**(6):631-648

Chapter 3

Modulating the Gut Microbiota to Combat Drug-Induced Liver Injury: A New Frontier in Hepatic Health

Ye Yang and Huikuan Chu

Abstract

Drug-induced liver injury (DILI) encompasses a spectrum of liver damage caused by pharmaceuticals or their metabolites, ranging from mild, asymptomatic liver dysfunction to severe, acute liver failure. The diagnosis of DILI primarily depends on a thorough understanding of its clinical presentation and the careful exclusion of alternative etiologies of liver injury. This chapter provides a comprehensive analysis of the epidemiology, pathogenesis, and therapeutic approaches to DILI, aiming to deepen the understanding of this complex condition. Furthermore, it investigates the emerging role of the gut microbiota in the pathogenesis of DILI, offering novel insights and potential avenues for future therapeutic interventions.

Keywords: drug-induced liver injury (DILI), drug-induced hepatitis, liver injury, gut microbiota, liver

1. Introduction

Drug-induced liver injury (DILI) refers to liver damage resulting from drugs and their metabolites [1], typically involving anti-infective agents, non-steroidal anti-inflammatory drugs (NSAIDs), psychotropic drugs, herbal remedies, dietary supplements, and anticancer agents. While the overall incidence of DILI remains relatively low, its frequency has increased in recent years, driven by the growing and diversifying global use of pharmaceuticals. Clinically, DILI manifests in various forms, including acute hepatitis, cholestasis, and, in severe cases, acute liver failure. In many Western countries, DILI is now the leading cause of acute liver failure, accounting for over half of all such cases [2]. The diagnosis of DILI remains challenging due to its nature as a diagnosis of exclusion and the absence of specific biomarkers. As a result, early recognition and management of DILI present significant difficulties for clinicians. A deeper understanding of the underlying factors and mechanisms of DILI is essential for advancing prevention and therapeutic strategies. Recent studies have underscored the pivotal role of gut microbiota in the pathogenesis of drug-induced liver injury [3]. The gut microbiota, a complex ecosystem of microorganisms inhabiting the human gastrointestinal tract, is integral to both the physiological and pathological processes of the liver. It influences energy metabolism, modulates immune responses, and contributes to pathogen defense. In addition to its role in liver diseases such as non-alcoholic fatty liver disease [4–7], alcoholic liver disease [8, 9], and hepatocellular carcinoma [10], gut microbiota also plays a critical role in the onset and progression of DILI. This article aims to provide a comprehensive analysis of the mechanisms through which gut microbiota contribute to drug-induced liver injury, thereby offering a scientific foundation for future research into the pathogenesis of DILI and the development of targeted prevention strategies.

2. Epidemiology

2.1 Global incidence

DILI represents a major cause of liver dysfunction worldwide. The global incidence of DILI is estimated to range between 13.9 and 24.0 cases per 100,000 individuals annually [11], although significant regional variations exist. In the United States, a comprehensive prospective study conducted by the U.S. Drug-Induced Liver injury Network (DILIN) reported an incidence of approximately 2.7 cases per 100,000 individuals [12]. In contrast, European nations exhibit higher rates, with Ireland reporting 19.1 cases per 100,000 [13], Spain at 3.42 [14], and France at 13.9 cases per 100,000 individuals annually [15].

In Asia, the widespread use of herbal medicines and dietary supplements (HDS) has been associated with an elevated incidence of DILI, particularly in China and South Korea. A national retrospective study conducted in China estimated the incidence at 23.8 cases per 100,000 individuals, which exceeds the rates observed in many Western countries [16] In South Korea, data from university hospitals indicate an incidence of approximately 12 cases per 100,000 individuals [17].

While data from Latin America and Africa remain limited, emerging studies suggest that the incidence of DILI in sub-Saharan Africa may be underreported, potentially due to inadequate access to medications and healthcare infrastructure [18]. Collectively, the global incidence of DILI is affected by various factors, including regional drug usage patterns, the maturity of health surveillance systems, and the effectiveness of adverse drug reaction reporting mechanisms.

2.2 High-risk groups of DILI

DILI exhibits variable incidence across different populations. It is notably more prevalent in certain groups, including the elderly, females, individuals with pre-existing chronic liver conditions, and those with specific genetic susceptibilities.

Older adults, particularly those aged 65 and older, represent a significant high-risk group for drug-induced liver injury, accounting for 33% of all reported cases [19]. Age-related declines in hepatic metabolic function lead to reduced drug clearance and increased drug accumulation, thereby heightening the risk of DILI [20]. Furthermore, polypharmacy is common in this population, with complex drug interactions and multidrug regimens further exacerbating the likelihood of liver injury [21]. In addition, genetic polymorphisms in drug metabolism, underlying liver disease, and individual variations in drug response play critical roles in determining susceptibility to DILI in elderly patients [22].

Gender significantly influences the pathogenesis of DILI, with women generally exhibiting a higher incidence than men. This disparity may be attributed to women's more pronounced immune responses, which could predispose them to immune-mediated liver damage upon drug exposure. Research suggests that women's immune systems react more vigorously to drug metabolites, thus increasing the likelihood of DILI [23]. In addition, sex hormones, particularly estrogen, play a crucial role in modulating the development of DILI in women. Estrogen influences the activity of hepatic enzymes, alters drug metabolism pathways, and enhances susceptibility to hepatotoxicity. Furthermore, sex-based differences in the activity of liver enzymes, such as Cytochrome P450 3A4 (CYP3A4)—which is often more active in women—may further modulate drug metabolism and DILI risk [24]. These gender-related differences may explain why women are more sensitive to certain medications, influencing both their metabolic response and the associated risk of liver injury.

Patients with chronic liver disease are particularly susceptible to DILI. Given that the liver is essential for drug metabolism, its impaired function in conditions such as cirrhosis or non-alcoholic fatty liver disease can compromise drug clearance and amplify hepatotoxicity. This risk is especially pronounced with drugs that are metabolized by the liver, including certain antibiotics, antiviral agents, and chemotherapy drugs. For example, patients with hepatitis B are 5.83 times more likely to develop DILI during anti-tuberculosis treatment compared to those without hepatitis B. Further analysis reveals that HBeAg-positive, immunotolerant patients are at a 2.10-fold increased risk of DILI relative to HBeAg-negative, inactive HBV carriers [25]. The degree of liver inflammation and fibrosis also plays a pivotal role in DILI susceptibility. In patients with non-alcoholic fatty liver disease, pre-existing liver inflammation, and steatosis significantly heighten the risk of drug-induced hepatotoxicity [26]. In advanced liver diseases, such as cirrhosis, the accumulation of drug metabolites may exacerbate liver damage, leading to more severe clinical manifestations [27]. Consequently, careful drug selection, dose adjustment, and vigilant monitoring of liver function are critical to mitigate DILI risk in this high-risk group.

Recent research has underscored the pivotal role of genetic factors in the susceptibility to DILI. Genetic predisposition influences both the metabolism of drugs and the liver's response to their toxicity. Variants in genes that regulate drug-metabolizing enzymes, receptors, or immune response pathways contribute to interindividual differences in drug responses. For example, polymorphisms within the cytochrome P450 (CYP450) enzyme family, essential for drug metabolism, are strongly associated with DILI. These genetic variations can lead to elevated drug concentrations in the body, thereby increasing hepatic stress and enhancing the risk of hepatotoxicity. Notably, Cytochrome P450 2D6 (CYP2D6) inhibitors have been shown to induce toxic reactions when co-administered with drugs such as metoprolol [28]. Additionally, specific human leukocyte antigen (HLA) genotypes, particularly HLA-B*5701, are closely linked to liver damage caused by certain medications, including antivirals [29]. Individuals carrying this allele are at a 60-fold higher risk of DILI compared to non-carriers, suggesting that particular immune genotypes may predispose individuals to drug-induced immune responses that contribute to liver injury [30]. Moreover, the antioxidant stress response in hepatocytes plays a critical role in modulating DILI. Polymorphisms in genes such as glutathione S-transferase mu 1 (GSTM1) and NAD(P)H quinone dehydrogenase 1 (NQO1) can alter the liver's ability to manage oxidative stress, making it more vulnerable to drug-induced oxidative damage, which further exacerbates hepatic injury [31].

3. Etiology

DILI results from exposure to a variety of substances, and more than 1000 drugs can cause DILI. With antibiotics, non-steroidal anti-inflammatory drugs (NSAIDs), antiepileptic drugs, herbal or dietary supplements, and anticancer drugs being among the most commonly implicated.

Antibiotic: Both prospective and retrospective studies have consistently identified anti-infective agents as a primary cause of DILI [32, 33]. A notable study by the DILIN in the United States found that antibiotics accounted for 45% of all DILI cases, with 408 out of 899 cases attributed to these drugs [34]. Among antibiotics, penicillins and cephalosporins were the most commonly implicated. In Ireland, amoxicillin-clavulanate emerged as the leading drug associated with DILI, with an incidence of approximately 43 cases per 100,000 users [35]. Similarly, data from China indicate that cephalosporins are the predominant antibiotics involved in DILI cases [36].

NSAIDs: NSAIDs are widely employed for their antipyretic and analgesic properties but can induce oxidative stress through the depletion of glutathione (GSH) and the production of reactive oxygen species (ROS), which in turn leads to hepatocellular necrosis and apoptosis [37–39]. Although the overall incidence of liver injury associated with NSAIDs is relatively low, typically 1 to 2 cases per 100,000 patients, the risk of DILI is notably higher in individuals with prolonged NSAID use or pre-existing liver conditions. Studies indicate that individuals aged over 75 are 5.7 times more likely to develop liver-related complications from NSAIDs compared to those under 45 [40]. Additionally, patients with underlying liver dysfunction are at increased risk of exacerbated hepatic injury when treated with NSAIDs [41].

Antiepileptic Drugs: The hepatotoxic potential of antiepileptic drugs, including valproic acid, carbamazepine, and phenytoin, is well-documented. Among these, valproic acid is the most frequently implicated, accounting for over 60% of DILI cases associated with antiepileptic medications. The risk of DILI typically peaks within the first 3 to 6 months of therapy with valproic acid, highlighting the necessity for regular liver function monitoring during this critical period to enable early detection of potential adverse effects [42]. Hepatic toxicity related to these drugs is frequently associated with mitochondrial dysfunction, which compounds the risk of severe liver damage.

Herbal and Dietary Supplements: The incidence of DILI associated with herbal and HDS has markedly increased in Asia in recent years, a trend largely driven by the growing use of these products, particularly in developing countries. In certain regions, herbal medicines and dietary supplements now contribute to a higher frequency of liver damage than conventional Western pharmaceuticals. Notably, substances such as turmeric, green tea extracts, and various herbal compounds have been frequently implicated in hepatotoxicity [43]. In Asia, the use of traditional Chinese herbs, including *Polygonum multiflorum*, is responsible for approximately 25% of all DILI cases [44]. As the consumption of herbal and dietary supplements continues to rise, the incidence of liver injuries linked to these substances is anticipated to increase further.

Anticancer Drugs: Anticancer agents are commonly associated with hepatotoxicity, which primarily arises from their direct intrinsic toxic effects. Liver injury is often manifested by elevated liver enzymes or bilirubin levels during treatment, but liver function typically normalizes following drug discontinuation or dose modification. This toxicity is generally dose-dependent and self-limiting, although in certain cases, it can progress to severe, chronic, or fatal liver damage. An analysis by Anna Pocurull et al. of patients with suspected drug-induced liver injury between 2018 and 2023 found that antitumor drugs accounted for 26% of all DILI cases, making them a predominant cause of hepatotoxicity in hospital settings [45].

4. Pathogenesis

The pathogenesis of drug-induced liver injury is complex and multifactorial, encompassing direct cellular toxicity, metabolic activation, and immune-mediated responses, each of which engages distinct molecular pathways that contribute to hepatic injury.

4.1 Activation of drug metabolism and production of reactive metabolites

Drugs are primarily metabolized in the liver via the cytochrome P450 enzyme system, a process that facilitates drug elimination [46]. However, this pathway also has a dual nature. In addition to promoting excretion, CYP450 metabolism can generate highly reactive metabolites, which may covalently interact with cellular macromolecules—such as proteins, DNA, and lipids—forming drug-protein adducts that provoke direct hepatotoxicity [47, 48]. For example, acetaminophen is metabolized in the liver to produce the reactive intermediate N-acetyl-p-benzoquinone imide (NAPQI), which induces mitochondrial oxidative stress by covalently modifying hepatocyte proteins. This results in DNA damage and subsequent hepatocyte necrosis [49]. Similarly, a range of other drugs, including certain antibiotics, antiviral agents, and chemotherapy agents, generate reactive metabolites through analogous metabolic pathways, thereby contributing to liver toxicity. Consequently, the formation of reactive metabolites during drug metabolism represents a critical mechanism underlying drug-induced liver injury, especially in individuals with pre-existing hepatic dysfunction.

4.2 Mitochondrial dysfunction

Certain drugs generate reactive metabolites during hepatic metabolism, which can impair the mitochondrial electron transport chain, leading to the accumulation of ROS and the onset of oxidative stress. A notable example is NAPQI, a toxic metabolite of acetaminophen (APAP), which uncouples oxidative phosphorylation (OXPHOS) and disrupts mitochondrial membrane potential [50]. This interference not only inhibits ATP synthesis but also damages mitochondrial complexes I and II, resulting in electron leakage and the generation of superoxide radicals [51]. Additionally, reduced mitochondrial membrane potential, a hallmark of DILI, may trigger the opening of the mitochondrial permeability transition pore (MPTP), further promoting hepatocyte apoptosis. For instance, cisplatin exacerbates liver damage by augmenting oxidative stress and compromising mitochondrial membrane potential [52]. Beyond oxidative stress, reactive drug metabolites can bind to mitochondrial DNA, causing mutations and functional impairment. The antiretroviral drug zidovudine (AZT) inhibits mitochondrial DNA replication by blocking DNA polymerase-γ, leading to a decrease in mitochondrial DNA copy number and mitochondrial dysfunction, thereby disrupting energy metabolism and inducing apoptosis [53]. Furthermore, mitochondrial autophagy, a critical process for maintaining mitochondrial quality control, can be hindered by drug-induced alterations in autophagic signaling pathways. In APAP-induced liver injury, for example, compromised mitochondrial autophagy is considered a pivotal step in the pathogenesis [54]. Finally, certain drugs can also impair cellular energy metabolism by inhibiting the tricarboxylic acid cycle and oxidative phosphorylation, thereby depleting energy reserves and contributing to hepatocyte death. Isoniazid, for example, targets mitochondrial respiratory complexes I-IV, significantly reducing the energy supply to liver cells and exacerbating liver injury [55].

4.3 Cholestasis and inhibition of bile salt effector protein (BSEP)

Drugs can impair bile secretion by inhibiting the Bile Salt Export Pump (BSEP), a critical transporter involved in hepatic bile acid efflux, thereby contributing to cholestatic liver injury [56–58]. Specifically, inhibition of BSEP leads to the accumulation of toxic bile acids within hepatocytes, which can induce cellular damage through apoptosis or necrosis. For example, cyclosporine A, a commonly prescribed immunosuppressant, directly interferes with BSEP function, disrupting bile salt transport and promoting the intracellular retention of bile acids. This retention triggers oxidative stress and activates inflammatory pathways, ultimately exacerbating cholestatic liver damage [59].

4.4 Immune-mediated liver injury

Recent studies have elucidated the intricate immunological mechanisms underlying immune-mediated DILI. This condition is characterized by hepatocyte damage, liver inflammation, and impaired liver function, resulting from the interaction between drugs or their metabolites and the host immune system. Drug-induced immune activation occurs through binding to cell surface receptors or endogenous liver proteins, triggering tissue damage [60]. The pathogenesis typically involves two key immune pathways: a T-cell-mediated response, in which the drug or its metabolites act as antigens on hepatocytes, and a B-cell-mediated response leading to antibody production. Additionally, DILI is often accompanied by the release of pro-inflammatory cytokines, such as TNF-α and IL-6, and the activation of macrophages and dendritic cells, further exacerbating the immune response [61]. In conclusion, immune-mediated drug-induced liver injury is a multifactorial process driven by several immune mechanisms. Future research should aim to elucidate the precise interactions between drugs and the immune system to inform the development of more targeted therapeutic and preventive strategies.

4.5 Genetic susceptibility

Drug-induced liver injury demonstrates considerable interindividual variability, primarily attributed to genetic differences in host susceptibility. Isoniazid (INH), a widely used anti-tuberculosis medication, is a prominent cause of DILI. Research has shown that polymorphisms in the N-acetyltransferase 2 (NAT2) gene significantly affect the metabolic rate of isoniazid, with slow acetylators exhibiting an increased risk of liver injury [62]. Similarly, genetic variations in Class I and Class II HLA genotypes have been identified as key factors influencing susceptibility to DILI induced by amoxicillin and clavulanate [63].

4.6 Impact of gut microbiota

Gut microbial imbalances are thought to exacerbate liver damage through mechanisms involving altered drug metabolism, enhanced inflammatory or oxidative stress responses, and dysregulation of hepatic immune functions, thereby accelerating the progression of liver pathology [64].

5. Conventional treatment approaches

DILI is a multifaceted clinical disorder characterized by a diverse array of etiologies and pathophysiological mechanisms. Consequently, available treatment strategies remain limited in scope and efficacy. Although current therapeutic approaches have yielded some improvements in patient outcomes, significant challenges, and unresolved issues continue to hinder optimal management.

5.1 Drug cessation

The cornerstone of managing DILI is the immediate discontinuation of the implicated drug(s) [65]. This intervention is critical for preventing continued liver damage and plays a pivotal role in arresting the progression of the injury. In the majority of cases, particularly among patients with mild hepatic impairment, cessation of the offending drug leads to the restoration of normal liver function [66].

5.2 Specific drug therapy

5.2.1 Detoxifying agents

N-Acetylcysteine (NAC) is a widely recognized therapeutic agent for acute liver injury resulting from acetaminophen overdose. Its mechanism of action involves the provision of cysteine, which facilitates the synthesis of glutathione and attenuates oxidative damage to hepatocytes [67].

Reduced glutathione is a vital intracellular metabolic regulator, renowned for its potent antioxidant activity. It plays a crucial role in maintaining the integrity of cellular and mitochondrial membranes, promotes hepatocyte regeneration, and accelerates the restoration of liver function [68]. Consequently, it is a pivotal therapeutic agent in the management of drug-induced liver injury.

5.2.2 Anti-inflammatory hepatoprotective agents

Bicyclic alcohols exert their therapeutic effects through multiple mechanisms, including the scavenging of reactive oxygen species, inhibition of lipid peroxidation, preservation of liver cell and mitochondrial membrane integrity, and suppression of inflammatory cytokine release. Collectively, these actions mitigate transaminase elevations associated with drug-induced hepatitis, thereby conferring hepatoprotection [69].

Silymarin, the primary active compound derived from *Silybum marianum* (milk thistle), exerts substantial effects through the inhibition of lipid peroxidation, scavenging of reactive oxygen species, stabilization of cell membranes, promotion of hepatocyte regeneration, and reduction of hyperlipidemia. Owing to its robust hepatoprotective properties, silymarin is extensively utilized in the clinical treatment of liver diseases, including hepatitis, cirrhosis, and drug-induced hepatic injury [70].

Glycyrrhetinic acid preparations, such as diammonium glycyrrhizinate, demonstrate potent anti-inflammatory properties and provide effective protection to liver cell membranes, thereby improving liver function. These compounds facilitate the repair of damaged hepatocytes and inhibit the release of pro-inflammatory mediators. Furthermore, glycyrrhetinic acid preparations stabilize cellular membranes, attenuate lipid peroxidation, and enhance hepatocyte resilience to toxic agents, collectively mitigating drug-induced liver injury [71].

Glucocorticoids represent a viable therapeutic option for DILI driven by immune-mediated mechanisms, including immune-mediated drug-induced hepatitis. Their efficacy is primarily attributed to the stabilization of lysosomal membranes, attenuation of non-specific bile duct inflammation, enhancement of bile flow, alleviation of systemic toxic responses, inhibition of antigen-antibody complex formation, and reduction of immune-mediated hepatocellular injury [72].

Polyene phosphatidylcholine, an essential constituent of cellular and subcellular membranes, is pivotal in liver cell regeneration, repair, and energy metabolism regulation. Additionally, it improves mitochondrial function within hepatocytes [73]. Given these properties, polyene phosphatidylcholine is considered a cornerstone in the treatment of DILI.

Thioprine, containing free thiol groups, serves to protect the structural integrity of liver mitochondria [74]. Additionally, it facilitates liver cell regeneration, scavenges reactive oxygen species, alleviates drug-induced toxicity [75], and significantly reduces liver damage in patients with DILI.

5.2.3 Choleretic agents

Ursodeoxycholic Acid (UDCA) is commonly employed in the management of cholestatic drug-induced liver injury, including that associated with antibiotics. It ameliorates liver damage induced by bile acids and inflammation through multiple mechanisms, including (i) preventing hepatocellular necrosis and apoptosis induced by bile acids, (ii) lowering bile acid levels and reducing their toxicity by promoting metabolic adaptations in hepatocytes, and (iii) exerting anti-inflammatory and immunomodulatory effects [76].

Adenosylmethionine functions as a methyl donor, modulating the methylation of liver cell membrane phospholipids, which alters membrane fluidity, promotes bile secretion, and prevents intrahepatic cholestasis. It also regulates hepatocyte regeneration and proliferation through the alanine transaminase pathway, thereby facilitating liver cell repair. Furthermore, adenosylmethionine is converted into cysteine, which is subsequently metabolized to produce glutathione, coenzyme A, and taurine. These metabolites enhance phospholipid biosynthesis in endothelial cells, stabilizing cellular structure and improving function. Additionally, adenosylmethionine augments the detoxification capacity of the bile acid metabolism system, reducing or preventing oxidative damage to hepatocytes induced by bile acid [77, 78].

5.3 Supportive therapy and clinical monitoring

For patients with severe DILI, discontinuation of the offending drug represents only the initial step in management. In addition to sustained supportive care to maintain fluid and electrolyte balance, rigorous monitoring is critical. This includes continuous assessment of liver function, coagulation status, renal function, and blood gas parameters to facilitate the early detection of liver failure and other complications. For patients requiring dialysis, liver support interventions, such as artificial liver support or liver transplantation, should be considered as part of a comprehensive therapeutic approach.

5.4 Liver transplantation

Liver transplantation is an established therapeutic option for end-stage liver disease and acute liver failure, frequently regarded as the last resort for patients with severe DILI, especially those progressing to acute liver failure [79]. However, despite its essential role in certain clinical scenarios, the broader application of liver transplantation is restricted by various limitations.

Although significant progress has been made in the treatment of DILI, considerable challenges persist. Current therapeutic approaches primarily involve discontinuing the causative drug and providing symptomatic support. However, in cases of severe liver injury, specific and targeted treatments remain unavailable. The pathogenesis of DILI is complex and multifactorial, involving pathways such as drug metabolites, oxidative stress, and immune-mediated mechanisms. Furthermore, substantial interindividual variability in response to treatment further limits the efficacy of current therapeutic strategies for the diverse spectrum of liver injuries.

6. A novel therapeutic approach for DILI: Targeting the intestinal microbiota

6.1 The role and physiological functions of the intestinal microbiota

The gut microbiota is a highly complex and diverse ecosystem, consisting of bacteria, fungi, viruses, and other microorganisms, which are widely distributed within the human gastrointestinal tract. This microbiota plays an essential role in digestion and metabolism. Notably, it ferments dietary fibers that are not absorbed in the small intestine, producing short-chain fatty acids (SCFAs) such as acetic acid, propionic acid, and butyric acid. These SCFAs not only provide energy to intestinal epithelial cells but also influence systemic metabolism through modulation of host metabolic pathways. Specifically, SCFAs activate G protein-coupled receptors like Free fatty acid receptor 3 (GPR41) and Free fatty acid receptor 2 (GPR43), which enhance energy metabolism, increase insulin sensitivity, lower blood glucose levels, and reduce the risk of non-alcoholic fatty liver disease [80]. Additionally, the gut microbiota affects bile acid metabolism, thereby regulating lipid absorption and maintaining cholesterol homeostasis [81].

Beyond its metabolic functions, the gut microbiota plays a critical role in immune regulation and maintaining intestinal barrier integrity, which is integral to the development of a range of diseases. In neuroendocrine disorders, for example, the microbiota produces neurotransmitters (e.g., serotonin) and other bioactive metabolites that regulate the gut-brain axis [82–84], influencing neural development and function. Moreover, by modulating the vagus nerve and the hypothalamic-pituitary-adrenal (HPA) axis, the gut microbiota can influence emotional and behavioral responses, with evidence linking dysbiosis to psychiatric conditions such as depression, anxiety, and autism [85]. In alcoholic fatty liver disease, pathogenic fungi such as *Candida albicans* contribute to liver fat accumulation and accelerate the progression of alcoholic liver disease through the TGF-β/let-7b-5p/Adrb3 pathway [8, 86]. In addition to fungi, specific gut bacteria also play a pivotal role in the progression and prognosis of ALD. For instance, *Enterococcus faecalis* exacerbates liver injury via TLR2 signaling, while the complement receptor CRIg on liver macrophages recognizes and clears *E. faecalis*, mitigating liver damage [9]. Furthermore, probiotics such as *Unclassified Coriobacteriaceae* and *Lactobacillus acidophilus* exert protective effects against alcoholic liver injury by modulating bile acid and phenylalanine metabolism, respectively [87, 88]. In obesity, an imbalance in the gut microbiota, particularly the ratio of Firmicutes to Bacteroidetes, is associated with increased energy intake and fat storage [89, 90]. Moreover, the gut microbiota plays a critical role in cancer pathogenesis and therapeutic responses, primarily through the modulation of immune and inflammatory pathways [91].

Recent studies have increasingly recognized the critical role of gut microbiota in DILI. A 2022 study, for example, reported that DILI patients exhibited lower levels of *Firmicutes* and *Bacteroidetes* at the phylum level, while *Proteobacteria* and *Actinobacteria* were found at elevated levels. At the genus level, *Bacteroides* and *Bifidobacterium* were significantly reduced in DILI patients [92]. This dysbiosis may be associated with the activation of the Nrf2 pathway by *B. longum* R0175, which reduces inflammation, mitigates oxidative stress, inhibits hepatocyte apoptosis, and restores microbial homeostasis, thereby alleviating acetaminophen-induced liver damage [93]. Furthermore, a separate study identified an increased abundance of lactic acid bacteria in patients with chronic DILI [94]. This shift may enhance the conversion of polyunsaturated fatty acids (PUFAs) into less toxic free saturated fatty acids, functioning as a negative feedback mechanism that partially counteracts the harmful effects of PUFA accumulation in DILI [92].

6.2 Mechanisms of gut microbiota in DILI

The specific mechanism by which gut microbiota regulates drug-induced liver injury may be as follows:

6.2.1 The role of gut barrier function and the gut-liver axis in DILI

The intestinal barrier is composed of physical, chemical, and immune components, including tight junction proteins, mucus layers, and immunoglobulin A (IgA), which collectively maintain homeostasis between the intestine and the liver. The gut microbiota plays a critical role in preserving the integrity of this barrier through the regulation of its various functions. Specifically, the microbiota promotes the expression of tight junction proteins, enhancing the intestinal epithelial barrier and preventing the translocation of harmful substances and pathogens into the bloodstream [95]. Furthermore, the gut microbiota secretes metabolites, such as SCFAs, that support the repair and regeneration of intestinal epithelial cells, thereby contributing to the overall stability of the intestinal barrier [96]. Dysbiosis of the gut microbiota compromises the intestinal barrier, leading to the translocation of bacterial toxins, including lipopolysaccharides (LPS), into the systemic circulation. This phenomenon, commonly referred to as "leaky gut," activates the Toll-like receptor 4 (TLR4) signaling pathway in the liver, triggering excessive Kupffer cell activation and initiating an inflammatory response [95, 97]. This cascade amplifies liver injury, positioning intestinal barrier dysfunction as a pivotal factor in the pathogenesis of DILI. The integrity of the intestinal barrier is intricately linked to the gut-liver axis. Dysregulation of this axis facilitates the entry of endotoxins into the bloodstream, which in turn activates the hepatic immune response and exacerbates liver damage [98]. Therefore, therapeutic strategies aimed at restoring microbial balance and regulating the gut-liver axis may provide a promising approach to mitigating drug-induced liver injury.

6.2.2 The key role of gut microbiota in drug metabolism

The gut microbiota plays a critical role in shaping drug metabolism, toxicity, and bioavailability. For example, Spanogiannopoulos et al. demonstrated through metabolomics that microbiota-derived enzymes can alter drug metabolites, thereby modulating both drug toxicity and the host's pharmacological response [99]. Similarly, Maier et al. reported that certain non-antibiotic medications can increase drug toxicity by reshaping the gut microbiota [100], particularly in individuals with high microbiota metabolic activity, who tend to have reduced drug tolerance and are more vulnerable to DILI. These findings highlight the potential of microbiota modulation as a strategy to reduce the production of toxic metabolites and mitigate the risk of DILI.

6.2.3 The role of gut microbiota in oxidative stress

Oxidative stress is a central mechanism in the pathogenesis of DILI, with the gut microbiota playing a pivotal role in its regulation. Ferrer et al. demonstrated that SCFAs produced by the gut microbiota can attenuate TNF-α-induced oxidative stress by modulating antioxidant enzyme activity [101]. Dysbiosis of the gut microbiota results in heightened oxidative stress and diminished hepatic antioxidant defenses, thereby exacerbating the progression of DILI. Therefore, therapeutic strategies aimed at modulating the gut microbiota to restore antioxidant homeostasis may represent a promising approach to mitigate DILI.

6.2.4 The regulation of hepatic immune system by gut microbiota

Recent studies have underscored the pivotal role of the gut microbiota in immune regulation, particularly in promoting the generation of regulatory T cells, which enhances immune tolerance and prevents autoimmune and excessive inflammatory responses [102]. Additionally, gut microbiota activate pattern recognition receptors, such as Toll-like receptors, to modulate innate immune responses and help the host defend against pathogen infections [97]. Consequently, the gut microbiota plays a crucial role in the development and regulation of the host immune system. DILI is often linked to excessive immune activation, highlighting the importance of gut microbiota in maintaining liver immune homeostasis. Llopis et al. demonstrated that gut microbiota imbalance increases endotoxin levels, triggering an overactive immune response in the liver, which exacerbates inflammation and liver damage [103]. Furthermore, recent research has revealed that microbial metabolites, including short-chain fatty acids and secondary bile acids, exert significant anti-inflammatory effects and are integral to regulating liver immune function [104]. Notably, the anaerobic, Gram-negative bacterium Akkermansia has been shown to alleviate oxidative stress and inflammation induced by acetaminophen. This bacterium enhances liver defense by restoring the balance between reduced and oxidized glutathione, increasing superoxide dismutase activity, and reducing the infiltration of pro-inflammatory immune cells and cytokines. In addition, Akkermansia contributes to liver immune balance by preserving intestinal barrier integrity, repairing disrupted gut microbiota, and promoting the production of short-chain fatty acids [105]. These findings emphasize the critical role of gut microbiota in liver immunity. Therefore, strategies aimed at modulating gut microbiota composition to restore liver immune balance offer promising therapeutic potential for DILI.

7. Potential therapeutic strategies based on gut microbiota modulation

The regulation of gut microbiota presents a promising therapeutic strategy for DILI. For example, anti-tuberculosis drugs can activate the TLR4-NF-κB-MyD88 signaling pathway, which contributes to liver damage. In contrast, high-dose *Lactobacillus casei* has been shown to suppress the activation of NF-κB and MyD88, thereby reducing oxidative stress and inflammation, and ultimately mitigating liver damage [106]. Moreover, propionic acid produced by gut microbiota has been demonstrated to protect C57BL/6 mice from liver injury induced by triptolide [107]. A meta-analysis by Xu et al. further confirmed that probiotics and prebiotics can significantly improve liver function by restoring gut microbiota balance [108]. Additionally, Wei Song et al. reported that oat-based postbiotics can alleviate liver injury, fatty acid metabolism dysfunction, and inflammation induced by a high-sucrose diet through the activation of the AMPK/SREBP-1c pathway, offering potential protective effects for DILI patients [109]. Collectively, these findings highlight that therapeutic approaches targeting gut microbiota regulation hold substantial promise, both in preclinical research and as potential clinical interventions for DILI.

8. Conclusion

DILI remains a prevalent and challenging condition in clinical practice. Current therapeutic approaches primarily focus on discontinuing the causative drug, alleviating hepatocellular damage, and implementing anti-inflammatory and antioxidant strategies. However, these interventions do not fully address the pathophysiological mechanisms underlying liver injury, and their effectiveness in improving long-term patient prognosis remains limited. Therefore, there is a pressing need for the development of more effective treatment options to enhance clinical outcomes.

In recent years, the significant role of gut microbiota in the pathogenesis of DILI has become increasingly evident. Gut microbiota influences liver injury both directly, by metabolizing drugs, and indirectly, through the regulation of intestinal barrier integrity and immune responses. These multifaceted interactions contribute to the onset and progression of DILI, positioning gut microbiota modulation as a promising therapeutic strategy.

As an emerging therapeutic target for DILI, gut microbiota provides valuable insights into the molecular mechanisms driving drug-induced liver injury and offers novel avenues for clinical intervention. Modulating gut microbiota may help mitigate liver damage by restoring microbial balance, reinforcing the intestinal barrier, and regulating immune responses. Future research should focus on elucidating the interactions between gut microbiota and DILI, with the aim of developing targeted interventions and evaluating their potential for clinical application.

Acknowledgements

We used ChatGPT to linguistically embellish the manuscript during its preparation to help improve the quality and clarity of its language.

Appendix and nomenclature

DILI	drug-induced liver injury
DILIN	drug-induced liver injury network
HDS	herbal medicines and dietary supplements
CYP450	cytochrome P450
NSAIDs	non-steroidal anti-inflammatory drugs
CYP3A4	cytochrome P450 3A4
HLA	human leukocyte antigen
GSTM1	glutathione S-transferase mu 1
NQO1	NAD(P)H quinone dehydrogenase 1
GSH	glutathione
NAPQI	N-acetyl-p-benzoquinone imide
CYP2D6	cytochrome P450 2D6
ROS	reactive oxygen species
OXPHOS	oxidative phosphorylation
MPTP	mitochondrial permeability transition pore
AZT	antiretroviral drug zidovudine
BSEP	bile salt export pump
NAT2	N-acetyltransferase 2
NAC	N-Acetylcysteine
UDCA	ursodeoxycholic acid
SCFAs	short-chain fatty acids
GPR41	free fatty acid receptor 3
GPR43	free fatty acid receptor 2
HPA	hypothalamic-pituitary-adrenal
PUFAs	polyunsaturated fatty acids
LPS	lipopolysaccharides
TLR4	toll-like receptor 4

Author details

Ye Yang[1] and Huikuan Chu[2*]

1 Union Hospital, Tongji Medical College, Huazhong University of Science and Technology, Wuhan, China

2 Division of Gastroenterology, Union Hospital, Tongji Medical College, Huazhong University of Science and Technology, Wuhan, China

*Address all correspondence to: 2012xh0827@hust.edu.cn

References

[1] David S, Hamilton JP. Drug-induced liver injury. US Gastroenterology & Hepatology Review. 2010;**6**:73-80

[2] Hoofnagle JH, Björnsson ES. Drug-induced liver injury - Types and phenotypes. The New England Journal of Medicine. 2019;**381**(3):264-273. DOI: 10.1056/NEJMra1816149

[3] Chen T, Li R, Chen P. Gut microbiota and chemical-induced acute liver injury. Frontiers in Physiology. 2021;**12**:688780. Published 2021 May 26. DOI: 10.3389/fphys.2021.688780

[4] Lee G, You HJ, Bajaj JS, et al. Distinct signatures of gut microbiome and metabolites associated with significant fibrosis in non-obese NAFLD. Nature Communications. 2020;**11**(1):4982. Published 2020 Oct 5. DOI: 10.1038/s41467-020-18754-5

[5] Demir M, Lang S, Hartmann P, et al. The fecal mycobiome in non-alcoholic fatty liver disease. Journal of Hepatology. 2022;**76**(4):788-799. DOI: 10.1016/j.jhep.2021.11.029

[6] Loomba R et al. Gut microbiome-based metagenomic signature for non-invasive detection of advanced fibrosis in human nonalcoholic fatty liver disease. Cell Metabolism. 2017;**25**(5):1054-1062.e5. DOI: 10.1016/j.cmet.2017.04.001

[7] Lang S et al. Intestinal virome signature associated with severity of nonalcoholic fatty liver disease. Gastroenterology. 2020;**159**(5):1839-1852. DOI: 10.1053/j.gastro.2020.07.005

[8] Chu H et al. The Candida albicans exotoxin candidalysin promotes alcohol-associated liver disease. Journal of Hepatology. 2020;**72**(3):391-400. DOI: 10.1016/j.jhep.2019.09.029

[9] Duan Y et al. CRIg on liver macrophages clears pathobionts and protects against alcoholic liver disease. Nature Communications. 2021;**12**(1):7172. DOI: 10.1038/s41467-021-27385-3

[10] Grąt M, Wronka KM, Krasnodębski M, et al. Profile of gut microbiota associated with the presence of hepatocellular cancer in patients with liver cirrhosis. Transplantation Proceedings. 2016;**48**(5):1687-1691. DOI: 10.1016/j.transproceed.2016.01.077

[11] Suk KT, Kim DJ. Drug-induced liver injury: Present and future. Clinical and Molecular Hepatology. 2012;**18**(3):249-257. DOI: 10.3350/cmh.2012.18.3.249

[12] Vega M, Verma M, Beswick D, et al. The incidence of drug- and herbal and dietary supplement-induced liver injury: Preliminary findings from gastroenterologist-based surveillance in the population of the State of Delaware. Drug Safety. 2017;**40**(9):783-787. DOI: 10.1007/s40264-017-0547-9

[13] Björnsson E. Review article: Drug-induced liver injury in clinical practice. Alimentary Pharmacology & Therapeutics. 2010;**32**(1):3-13. DOI: 10.1111/j.1365-2036.2010.04320.x

[14] Andrade RJ, Lucena MI, Fernández MC, et al. Drug-induced liver injury: An analysis of 461 incidences submitted to the Spanish registry over a 10-year period [published correction appears in Gastroenterology. 2005 Nov;129(5):1808]. Gastroenterology. 2005;**129**(2):512-521. DOI: 10.1016/j.gastro.2005.05.006

[15] Sgro C, Clinard F, Ouazir K, et al. Incidence of drug-induced hepatic injuries: A French population-based study. Hepatology. 2002;**36**(2):451-455. DOI: 10.1053/jhep.2002.34857

[16] Shen T, Liu Y, Shang J, et al. Incidence and etiology of drug-induced liver injury in mainland China. Gastroenterology. 2019;**156**(8):2230-2241.e11. DOI: 10.1053/j.gastro.2019.02.002

[17] Suk KT, Kim DJ, Kim CH, et al. A prospective nationwide study of drug-induced liver injury in Korea. The American Journal of Gastroenterology. 2012;**107**(9):1380-1387. DOI: 10.1038/ajg.2012.138

[18] Riebensahm C et al. A closer look at the spectrum of drug-induced liver injury in sub-Saharan Africa. Expert Review of Clinical Pharmacology. 2019;**12**(9):875-883. DOI: 10.1080/17512433.2019.1638251

[19] Weersink RA, Alvarez-Alvarez I, Medina-Cáliz I, et al. Clinical characteristics and outcome of drug-induced liver injury in the older patients: From the young-old to the oldest-old. Clinical Pharmacology and Therapeutics. 2021;**109**(4):1147-1158. DOI: 10.1002/cpt.2108

[20] Woodhouse K. Drugs and the liver. Part III: Ageing of the liver and the metabolism of drugs. Biopharmaceutics & Drug Disposition. 1992;**13**(5):311-320. DOI: 10.1002/bdd.2510130502

[21] Maddrey WC. Drug-induced hepatotoxicity: 2005. Journal of Clinical Gastroenterology. 2005;**39**(4 Suppl. 2):S83-S89. DOI: 10.1097/01.mcg.0000155548.91524.6e

[22] George N, Chen M, Yuen N, Hunt CM, Suzuki A. Interplay of gender, age and drug properties on reporting frequency of drug-induced liver injury. Regulatory Toxicology and Pharmacology. 2018;**94**:101-107. DOI: 10.1016/j.yrtph.2018.01.018

[23] Amacher DE. Female gender as a susceptibility factor for drug-induced liver injury. Human & Experimental Toxicology. 2014;**33**(9):928-939. DOI: 10.1177/0960327113512860

[24] Parkinson A, Mudra DR, Johnson C, Dwyer A, Carroll KM. The effects of gender, age, ethnicity, and liver cirrhosis on cytochrome P450 enzyme activity in human liver microsomes and inducibility in cultured human hepatocytes. Toxicology and Applied Pharmacology. 2004;**199**(3):193-209. DOI: 10.1016/j.taap.2004.01.010

[25] Zheng YX, Ma SJ, Tan DM, et al. Meta-analysis of liver injury during anti-tuberculosis treatment in patients with hepatitis B. Chinese Journal of Hepatology. 2014;**22**(8):585-589. DOI: 10.3760/cma.j.issn.1007-3418.2014.08.007

[26] Lammert C, Imler T, Teal E, Chalasani N. Patients with chronic liver disease suggestive of nonalcoholic fatty liver disease may be at higher risk for drug-induced liver injury. Clinical Gastroenterology and Hepatology. 2019;**17**(13):2814-2815. DOI: 10.1016/j.cgh.2018.12.013

[27] Dietrich CG, Götze O, Geier A. Molecular changes in hepatic metabolism and transport in cirrhosis and their functional importance. World Journal of Gastroenterology. 2016;**22**(1):72-88. DOI: 10.3748/wjg.v22.i1.72

[28] Bahar MA, Kamp J, Borgsteede SD, Hak E, Wilffert B. The impact of CYP2D6 mediated drug-drug interaction: A systematic review on a combination of metoprolol and paroxetine/fluoxetine.

British Journal of Clinical Pharmacology. 2018;**84**(12):2704-2715. DOI: 10.1111/bcp.13741

[29] Daly AK. Using genome-wide association studies to identify genes important in serious adverse drug reactions. Annual Review of Pharmacology and Toxicology. 2012;**52**:21-35. DOI: 10.1146/annurev-pharmtox-010611-134743

[30] Mallal S, Phillips E, Carosi G, et al. HLA-B*5701 screening for hypersensitivity to abacavir. The New England Journal of Medicine. 2008;**358**(6):568-579. DOI: 10.1056/NEJMoa0706135

[31] Zhu Y, Yang JH, Hu JP, Qiao M. Association of glutathione S-transferases (GSTT1, GSTM1 and GSTP1) genes polymorphisms with nonalcoholic fatty liver disease susceptibility: A PRISMA-compliant systematic review and meta-analysis. Medicine (Baltimore). 2022;**101**(38):e30803. DOI: 10.1097/MD.0000000000030803

[32] Björnsson E, Olsson R. Outcome and prognostic markers in severe drug-induced liver disease. Hepatology. 2005;**42**(2):481-489. DOI: 10.1002/hep.20800

[33] Chalasani N, Fontana RJ, Bonkovsky HL, et al. Causes, clinical features, and outcomes from a prospective study of drug-induced liver injury in the United States. Gastroenterology. 2008;**135**(6):1924-1934.e19344. DOI: 10.1053/j.gastro.2008.09.011

[34] Chalasani N, Bonkovsky HL, Fontana R, et al. Features and outcomes of 899 patients with drug-induced liver injury: The DILIN prospective study. Gastroenterology. 2015;**148**(7):1340-52.e7. DOI: 10.1053/j.gastro.2015.03.006

[35] Björnsson ES, Bergmann OM, Björnsson HK, Kvaran RB, Olafsson S. Incidence, presentation, and outcomes in patients with drug-induced liver injury in the general population of Iceland. Gastroenterology. 2013;**144**(7):1419-1e20. DOI: 10.1053/j.gastro.2013.02.006

[36] Kong XH, Guo DH, Yao C, Yang HY, Liu SY, Yu CX, et al. Active monitoring of drug-induced liver injury in 156,570 hospitalized patients using an information system. Herald of Medicine. 2021;**40**(4):472-477

[37] Jadeja RN, Urrunaga NH, Dash S, Khurana S, Saxena NK. Withaferin-A reduces acetaminophen-induced liver injury in mice. Biochemical Pharmacology. 2015;**97**(1):122-132. DOI: 10.1016/j.bcp.2015.07.024

[38] Song E, Fu J, Xia X, Su C, Song Y. Bazhen decoction protects against acetaminophen induced acute liver injury by inhibiting oxidative stress, inflammation and apoptosis in mice. PLoS One. 2014;**9**(9):e107405. Published 2014 Sep 15. DOI: 10.1371/journal.pone.0107405

[39] Ramachandran A, Jaeschke H. Mechanisms of acetaminophen hepatotoxicity and their translation to the human pathophysiology. Journal of Clinical and Translational Research. 2017;**3**(Suppl. 1):157-169. DOI: 10.18053/jctres.03.2017S1.002

[40] Bessone F. Non-steroidal anti-inflammatory drugs: What is the actual risk of liver damage? World Journal of Gastroenterology. 2010;**16**(45):5651-5661. DOI: 10.3748/wjg.v16.i45.5651

[41] Soleimanpour M, Imani F, Safari S, et al. The role of non-steroidal anti-inflammatory drugs (NSAIDs) in the treatment of patients with hepatic disease: A review article. Anesthesiology

and Pain Medicine. 2016;**6**(4):e37822. Published 2016 Aug 10. DOI: 10.5812/aapm.37822

[42] Hope B, Syed-Mohammed J, Ahmed E. S3281 a rare case of drug-induced liver injury (DILI) due to valproate hepatocellular injury. The American Journal of Gastroenterology. 2022;**117**(10S):pe2087-pe2088. DOI: 10.14309/01.ajg.0000869764.60904.0b

[43] Patel-Rodrigues PA, Cundra L, Alhaqqan D, Gildea DT, Woo SM, Lewis JH. Herbal- and dietary-supplement-induced liver injury: A review of the recent literature. Liver. 2024;**4**(1):94-118. DOI: 10.3390/livers4010008

[44] Byeon JH, Kil JH, Ahn YC, Son CG. Systematic review of published data on herb induced liver injury. Journal of Ethnopharmacology. 2019;**233**:190-196. DOI: 10.1016/j.jep.2019.01.006

[45] Pocurull A, Moreta MJ, Heitman D, et al. Anticancer drugs are the first cause of drug-induced liver injury in a reference hospital. Liver International. 2024;**44**(2):286-292. DOI: 10.1111/liv.15821

[46] Zhao M, Ma J, Li M, et al. Cytochrome P450 enzymes and drug metabolism in humans. International Journal of Molecular Sciences. 2021;**22**(23):12808. Published 2021 Nov 26. DOI: 10.3390/ijms222312808

[47] Villanueva-Paz M, Morán L, López-Alcántara N, et al. Oxidative stress in drug-induced liver injury (DILI): From mechanisms to biomarkers for use in clinical practice. Antioxidants (Basel). 2021;**10**(3):390. Published 2021 Mar 5. DOI: 10.3390/antiox10030390

[48] Hughes TB, Flynn N, Dang NL, Swamidass SJ. Modeling the bioactivation and subsequent reactivity of Drugs. Chemical Research in Toxicology. 2021;**34**(2):584-600. DOI: 10.1021/acs.chemrestox.0c00417

[49] Jaeschke H, McGill MR, Ramachandran A. Oxidant stress, mitochondria, and cell death mechanisms in drug-induced liver injury: Lessons learned from acetaminophen hepatotoxicity. Drug Metabolism Reviews. 2012;**44**(1):88-106. DOI: 10.3109/03602532.2011.602688

[50] Moles A, Torres S, Baulies A, Garcia-Ruiz C, Fernandez-Checa JC. Mitochondrial-lysosomal axis in acetaminophen hepatotoxicity. Frontiers in Pharmacology. 2018;**9**:453. Published 2018 May 15. DOI: 10.3389/fphar.2018.00453

[51] Jaeschke H, McGill MR, Ramachandran A. Oxidant stress, mitochondria, and cell death mechanisms in drug-induced liver injury: Lessons learned from acetaminophen hepatotoxicity. Drug Metabolism Reviews. 2012;**44**(1):88-106. DOI: 10.3109/03602532.2011.602688

[52] Han W, Jianhua C, Shili S, et al. Inhibition effect of hydrogen water on cisplatin induced hepatocyte injury via upregulating NFE2L2/HMOX1 expression[J]. Chinese General Practice. DOI: 10.12114/j.issn.1007-9572.2024.0093

[53] Santos-Llamas A, Monte MJ, Marin JJG, Perez MJ. Dysregulation of autophagy in rat liver with mitochondrial DNA depletion induced by the nucleoside analogue zidovudine. Archives of Toxicology. 2018;**92**(6):2109-2118. DOI: 10.1007/s00204-018-2200-5

[54] Pan M, Shi XY. The role of mitophagy in the occurrence and

development of liver-related diseases. Journal of Clinical Hepatobiliary Diseases. 2024;**40**(2):413-418

[55] Nhung TTM, Phat NK, Nghi TD, et al. Endoplasmic reticulum stress inhibition preserves mitochondrial function and cell survival during early onset of isoniazid-induced oxidative stress. bioRxiv. DOI: 10.1101/2024.08.12.607527

[56] Kenna JG et al. Can bile salt export pump inhibition testing in drug discovery and development reduce liver injury risk? An international transporter consortium perspective. Clinical Pharmacology and Therapeutics. 2018;**104**(5):916-932. DOI: 10.1002/cpt.1222

[57] Dawson S et al. In vitro inhibition of the bile salt export pump correlates with risk of cholestatic drug-induced liver injury in humans. Drug Metabolism and Disposition: The Biological Fate of Chemicals. 2012;**40**(1):130-138. DOI: 10.1124/dmd.111.040758

[58] Morgan RE et al. Interference with bile salt export pump function is a susceptibility factor for human liver injury in drug development. Toxicological Sciences : An Official Journal of the Society of Toxicology. 2010;**118**(2):485-500. DOI: 10.1093/toxsci/kfq269

[59] Stieger B, Fattinger K, Madon J, Kullak-Ublick GA, Meier PJ. Drug- and estrogen-induced cholestasis through inhibition of the hepatocellular bile salt export pump (Bsep) of rat liver. Gastroenterology. 2000;**118**(2):422-430. DOI: 10.1016/s0016-5085(00)70224-1

[60] Gerussi A et al. Immune-mediated drug-induced liver injury: Immunogenetics and experimental models. International Journal of Molecular Sciences. 2021;**22**(9):4557. DOI: 10.3390/ijms22094557

[61] Gerussi A, Natalini A, Antonangeli F, et al. Immune-mediated drug-induced liver injury: Immunogenetics and experimental models. International Journal of Molecular Sciences. 2021;**22**(9):4557. Published 2021 Apr 27. DOI: 10.3390/ijms22094557

[62] Yoon JG, Jang DG, Cho SG, et al. Synergistic toxicity with copper contributes to NAT2-associated isoniazid toxicity. Experimental & Molecular Medicine. 2024;**56**(3):570-582. DOI: 10.1038/s12276-024-01172-8

[63] Lucena MI, Molokhia M, Shen Y, et al. Susceptibility to amoxicillin-clavulanate-induced liver injury is influenced by multiple HLA class I and II alleles. Gastroenterology. 2011;**141**(1):338-347. DOI: 10.1053/j.gastro.2011.04.001

[64] Li G et al. Interplay between drug-induced liver injury and gut microbiota: A comprehensive overview. Cellular and Molecular Gastroenterology and Hepatology. 2024;**18**(3):101355. DOI: 10.1016/j.jcmgh.2024.05.003

[65] Li M et al. Pharmacotherapies for drug-induced liver injury: A current literature review. Frontiers in Pharmacology. 2022;**12**:806249. DOI: 10.3389/fphar.2021.806249

[66] Devarbhavi H et al. Single-center experience with drug-induced liver injury from India: Causes, outcome, prognosis, and predictors of mortality. The American Journal of Gastroenterology. 2010;**105**(11):2396-2404. DOI: 10.1038/ajg.2010.287

[67] Licata A, Minissale MG, Stankevičiūtė S, et al. N-Acetylcysteine for preventing acetaminophen-induced

liver injury: A comprehensive review. Frontiers in Pharmacology. 2022;**13**:828565. Published 2022 Aug 10. DOI: 10.3389/fphar.2022.828565

[68] Elsawy H et al. Naringin alleviates methotrexate-induced liver injury in male albino rats and enhances its antitumor efficacy in HepG2 cells. Bioscience Reports. 2020;**40**(6):BSR20193686. DOI: 10.1042/BSR20193686

[69] Wang Y, Lai R, Zong P, et al. Bicyclol for the treatment of drug-induced liver injury: A propensity score matching analysis using a nationwide inpatient database. The Journal of International Medical Research. 2021;**49**(4):3000605211005945. DOI: 10.1177/03000605211005945

[70] Zhang J, Xi J, He R, Pan J, Zhuang S, Zhao Y, et al. Experimental study on the hepatoprotective effects of silymarin derivatives. Chinese Journal of Traditional Medical Science and Technology. 2024;**31**(6):988-991

[71] Lu F, Li Z, Pan W, He J. Protective effect of diammoniuni glycyrrhizinate injection combined with salvia injection on acute liver injury induced by CC14 in mice. Traditional Chinese Drug Research and Clinical Pharmacology. 2020;**31**(7):810-814

[72] Liu Y, Guo Y, Xu H, Feng H, Chen D, Pan F. Current application of glucocorticoids in drug-induced liver injury. Chinese Journal of Integrated Traditional and Western Medicine on Liver Diseases. 2024;**34**(6):562-565

[73] Leng N, Liu Y, Qiu Y, Jiang F, Fu S, Wei S, et al. Network meta analysis of five liver protective drugs in the treatment of drug-induced liver injury. China Medicine and Pharmacy. 2022;**12**(8):42-47106

[74] Zhang J, Xi J, He R, et al. Experimental study on the hepatoprotective effects of silymarin derivatives. China Journal of Traditional Chinese Medicine and Pharmacy. 2024;**31**:988-991

[75] Yu J, Hu L, Wu ZY. Analysis of the efficacy of tiopronin combined with bisoprolol in the treatment of hepatitis B. Journal of Laboratory Medicine and Clinical Sciences. 2020;**17**:3660-3662

[76] Razori MV et al. Anticholestatic mechanisms of ursodeoxycholic acid in lipopolysaccharide-induced cholestasis. Biochemical Pharmacology. 2019;**168**:48-56. DOI: 10.1016/j.bcp.2019.06.009

[77] Xiao L, Hu X, Cai YK, et al. Efficacy of adenosylmethionine combined with reduced glutathione in the treatment of drug-induced liver injury. Practical Hepatology Journal. 2022;**25**:66-69

[78] Mullins C et al. Drug-induced liver injury (DILI) with Micafungin: The importance of causality assessment. The Annals of Pharmacotherapy. 2020;**54**(6):526-532. DOI: 10.1177/1060028019892587

[79] Wang Y, Liang Y. Progress in liver transplantation for drug-induced liver injury. Organ Transplantation. 2022;**13**(03):338-343

[80] Zhang S, Zhao J, Xie F, et al. Dietary fiber-derived short-chain fatty acids: A potential therapeutic target to alleviate obesity-related nonalcoholic fatty liver disease. Obesity Reviews. 2021;**22**(11):e13316. DOI: 10.1111/obr.13316

[81] Sayin SI, Wahlström A, Felin J, et al. Gut microbiota regulates bile acid metabolism by reducing the levels of tauro-beta-muricholic acid, a naturally occurring FXR antagonist.

Cell Metabolism. 2013;**17**(2):225-235. DOI: 10.1016/j.cmet.2013.01.003

[82] Gao K, Pi Y, Mu CL, Farzi A, Liu Z, Zhu WY. Increasing carbohydrate availability in the hindgut promotes hypothalamic neurotransmitter synthesis: Aromatic amino acids linking the microbiota-brain axis. Journal of Neurochemistry. 2019;**149**(5):641-659. DOI: 10.1111/jnc.14709

[83] Lukić I, Getselter D, Koren O, Elliott E. Role of tryptophan in microbiota-induced depressive-like behavior: Evidence from tryptophan depletion study. Frontiers in Behavioral Neuroscience. 2019;**13**:123. Published 2019 Jun 4. DOI: 10.3389/fnbeh.2019.00123

[84] Gao K, Pi Y, Mu CL, Peng Y, Huang Z, Zhu WY. Antibiotics-induced modulation of large intestinal microbiota altered aromatic amino acid profile and expression of neurotransmitters in the hypothalamus of piglets. Journal of Neurochemistry. 2018;**146**(3):219-234. DOI: 10.1111/jnc.14333

[85] Socała K, Doboszewska U, Szopa A, et al. The role of microbiota-gut-brain axis in neuropsychiatric and neurological disorders. Pharmacological Research. 2021;**172**:105840. DOI: 10.1016/j.phrs.2021.105840

[86] Zhao J et al. Hepatocyte TGF-β signaling inhibiting WAT browning to promote NAFLD and obesity is associated with let-7b-5p. Hepatology Communications. 2022;**6**(6):1301-1321. DOI: 10.1002/hep4.1892

[87] Chu H, Jiang L, Gao B, et al. The selective PPAR-delta agonist seladelpar reduces ethanol-induced liver disease by restoring gut barrier function and bile acid homeostasis in mice. Translational Research. 2021;**227**:1-14. DOI: 10.1016/j.trsl.2020.06.006

[88] Chen L et al. Modulating phenylalanine metabolism by L. acidophilus alleviates alcohol-related liver disease through enhancing intestinal barrier function. Cell & Bioscience. 2023;**13**(1):24. DOI: 10.1186/s13578-023-00974-z

[89] Krajmalnik-Brown R, Ilhan ZE, Kang DW, DiBaise JK. Effects of gut microbes on nutrient absorption and energy regulation. Nutrition in Clinical Practice. 2012;**27**(2):201-214. DOI: 10.1177/0884533611436116

[90] Magne F, Gotteland M, Gauthier L, et al. The firmicutes/bacteroidetes ratio: A relevant marker of gut dysbiosis in obese patients? Nutrients. 2020;**12**(5):1474. Published 2020 May 19. DOI: 10.3390/nu12051474

[91] Xue M, Liang H, Ji X, et al. Effects of fucoidan on gut flora and tumor prevention in 1,2-dimethylhydrazine-induced colorectal carcinogenesis. The Journal of Nutritional Biochemistry. 2020;**82**:108396. DOI: 10.1016/j.jnutbio.2020.108396

[92] Zhao S, Fu H, Zhou T, et al. Alteration of bile acids and omega-6 PUFAs are correlated with the progression and prognosis of drug-induced liver injury. Frontiers in Immunology. 2022;**13**:772368. Published 2022 Apr 12. DOI: 10.3389/fimmu.2022.772368

[93] Li S, Zhuge A, Xia J, et al. Bifidobacterium longum R0175 protects mice against APAP-induced liver injury by modulating the Nrf2 pathway. Free Radical Biology & Medicine. 2023;**203**:11-23. DOI: 10.1016/j.freeradbiomed.2023.03.026

[94] Liu B, Zeng Q, Chen H, et al. The hepatotoxicity of altrazine exposure in mice involves the intestinal microbiota.

Chemosphere. 2021;**272**:129572. DOI: 10.1016/j.chemosphere.2021.129572

[95] Gong HY, Wu JX, Yang XY, et al. Advances in research on the antiviral mechanisms of gut microbiota. Acta Veterinaria et Zootechnica Sinica. 2023;**54**(12):4910-4919

[96] Pearce SC, Weber GJ, van Sambeek DM, Soares JW, Racicot K, Breault DT. Intestinal enteroids recapitulate the effects of short-chain fatty acids on the intestinal epithelium. PLoS One. 2020;**15**(4):e0230231. Published 2020 Apr 2. DOI: 10.1371/journal.pone.0230231

[97] Hug H, Mohajeri MH, La Fata G. Toll-like receptors: Regulators of the immune response in the human gut. Nutrients. 2018;**10**(2):203. Published 2018 Feb 13. DOI: 10.3390/nu10020203

[98] Tripathi A, Debelius J, Brenner DA, et al. The gut-liver axis and the intersection with the microbiome [published correction appears in Nat Rev Gastroenterol Hepatol. 2018 Dec;15(12):785. Doi: 10.1038/s41575-018-0031-8]. Nature Reviews. Gastroenterology & Hepatology. 2018;**15**(7):397-411. DOI: 10.1038/s41575-018-0011-z

[99] Spanogiannopoulos P, Bess EN, Carmody RN, Turnbaugh PJ. The microbial pharmacists within us: A metagenomic view of xenobiotic metabolism. Nature Reviews. Microbiology. 2016;**14**(5):273-287. DOI: 10.1038/nrmicro.2016.17

[100] Maier L, Pruteanu M, Kuhn M, et al. Extensive impact of non-antibiotic drugs on human gut bacteria. Nature. 2018;**555**(7698):623-628. DOI: 10.1038/nature25979

[101] Ferrer M, Buey B, Grasa L, Mesonero JE, Latorre E. Protective role of short-chain fatty acids on intestinal oxidative stress induced by TNF-α. Cell Stress Chaperones. 2024;**29**(6):769-776. DOI: 10.1016/j.cstres.2024.11.002

[102] Yao X, Zhang C, Xing Y, et al. Remodelling of the gut microbiota by hyperactive NLRP3 induces regulatory T cells to maintain homeostasis. Nature Communications. 2017;**8**(1):1896. Published 2017 Dec 1. DOI: 10.1038/s41467-017-01917-2

[103] Llopis M, Cassard AM, Wrzosek L, et al. Intestinal microbiota contributes to individual susceptibility to alcoholic liver disease. Gut. 2016;**65**(5):830-839. DOI: 10.1136/gutjnl-2015-310585

[104] Visekruna A, Luu M. The role of short-chain fatty acids and bile acids in intestinal and liver function, inflammation, and carcinogenesis. Frontiers in Cell and Development Biology. 2021;**9**:703218. Published 2021 Jul 26. DOI: 10.3389/fcell.2021.703218

[105] Huang Y, Zhang Y, Wu K, Tan X, Lan T, Wang G. Role of gut microecology in the pathogenesis of drug-induced liver injury and emerging therapeutic strategies. Molecules. 2024;**29**(11):2663. Published 2024 Jun 4. DOI: 10.3390/molecules29112663

[106] Li Y, Zhao L, Sun C, et al. Regulation of gut microflora by *Lactobacillus casei* Zhang attenuates liver injury in mice caused by anti-tuberculosis drugs. International Journal of Molecular Sciences. 2023;**24**(11):9444. Published 2023 May 29. DOI: 10.3390/ijms24119444

[107] Huang JF, Zhao Q, Dai MY, et al. Gut microbiota protects from triptolide-induced hepatotoxicity: Key role of propionate and its downstream signalling events. Pharmacological Research. 2020;**155**:104752. DOI: 10.1016/j.phrs.2020.104752

[108] Xu S, Zhao M, Wang Q, et al. Effectiveness of probiotics and prebiotics against acute liver injury: A meta-analysis. Frontiers in Medicine (Lausanne). 2021;**8**:739337. Published 2021 Sep 21. DOI: 10.3389/fmed.2021.739337

[109] Song W, Wen R, Liu T, et al. Oat-based postbiotics ameliorate high-sucrose induced liver injury and colitis susceptibility by modulating fatty acids metabolism and gut microbiota. The Journal of Nutritional Biochemistry. 2024;**125**:109553. DOI: 10.1016/j.jnutbio.2023.109553

Chapter 4

Dual-Energy Computed Tomography for the Evaluation of Amiodarone-Induced Hepatotoxicity

Hongwei Zhao, Hu Liu and Haijuan Lv

Abstract

Amiodarone is a widely used antiarrhythmic drug, particularly effective for treating various cardiac arrhythmias. However, prolonged use of amiodarone is associated with hepatotoxicity, primarily due to iodine accumulation in the liver, which can range from asymptomatic enzyme elevation to severe liver injury. Traditional diagnostic methods, such as liver function tests and single-energy computed tomography (CT) scans, have limitations in accurately detecting and quantifying iodine accumulation, especially in the presence of conditions like hepatic steatosis. Dual-energy computed tomography (DECT) has emerged as a promising non-invasive diagnostic tool that provides a more accurate assessment of hepatic iodine concentration, overcoming many limitations of conventional imaging. This chapter explores the application of DECT in quantifying iodine deposition in patients undergoing long-term amiodarone therapy, enabling early detection of hepatotoxicity and facilitating individualized treatment plans. The use of DECT not only allows for precise monitoring of hepatic changes but also offers a potential non-invasive biomarker for managing amiodarone-induced hepatotoxicity, enhancing patient safety, and improving clinical outcomes.

Keywords: amiodarone, hepatotoxicity, dual-energy computed tomography, iodine accumulation, non-invasive diagnosis, liver function

1. Introduction

Amiodarone is one of the most widely used antiarrhythmic drugs in clinical practice, particularly valued for its effectiveness in managing diverse cardiac arrhythmias, including atrial fibrillation and ventricular tachycardia [1]. This drug's complex pharmacological profile, which includes potassium channel blockade, among other mechanisms, enhances its broad antiarrhythmic properties and accounts for its extensive use in reducing arrhythmic events and improving survival rates in patients with high-risk arrhythmias.

Despite these therapeutic benefits, long-term use of amiodarone has been associated with significant adverse effects, most notably hepatotoxicity. Clinical studies indicate that between 15 and 50% of patients on chronic amiodarone therapy experience hepatotoxicity, ranging from asymptomatic liver enzyme elevations to severe liver injury and, in rare cases, acute liver failure [2]. This hepatotoxic effect is largely attributed to the drug's high iodine content; amiodarone is an iodinated benzofuran derivative, and its iodine accumulates within the liver over time. Studies involving animal models confirm that after approximately 2 months of amiodarone administration, liver iodine levels can increase six to tenfold [3]. This excessive iodine buildup has been associated with cellular toxicity, oxidative stress, and inflammatory responses, ultimately impairing liver function. Early detection of amiodarone-induced hepatotoxicity is crucial to prevent progression to severe liver damage and to allow timely interventions, such as dose adjustment or drug discontinuation.

Traditional methods for monitoring hepatotoxicity, such as liver enzyme tests and single-energy CT scans, present limitations when assessing hepatic iodine accumulation. While elevated liver CT attenuation values may correlate with iodine concentration, they may not provide a reliable assessment in patients with other concurrent liver conditions, such as hepatic steatosis, that alter CT attenuation. Such cases may lead to either underestimation or overestimation of hepatic changes. Moreover, conventional CT cannot effectively differentiate between different causes of elevated liver density, such as iron overload in conditions like hemochromatosis and hemosiderosis.

Dual-energy computed tomography (DECT) emerges as a promising imaging modality that overcomes these limitations by using two different energy spectra to obtain images. This dual-energy approach enables material decomposition based on the distinct attenuation properties of tissues at varying energy levels, allowing for accurate, non-invasive quantification of iodine concentration in the liver. DECT thus provides a more reliable assessment of hepatic iodine deposition, irrespective of other concurrent hepatic conditions [4].

By distinguishing iodine from other substances in the liver, DECT enables precise detection and quantification of hepatic iodine accumulation associated with amiodarone therapy. This technology offers a valuable tool for the early diagnosis and monitoring of hepatotoxicity, facilitating timely clinical decision-making and potentially improving outcomes for patients receiving long-term amiodarone treatment.

2. Pathophysiology of amiodarone-induced hepatotoxicity

Amiodarone is a commonly used antiarrhythmic drug, but its use can lead to hepatotoxicity characterized by elevated liver enzymes and potential liver damage. The pathophysiology of amiodarone-induced hepatotoxicity is multifactorial, with the accumulation of iodine in the liver playing a crucial role.

2.1 Iodine accumulation

Amiodarone contains a large amount of iodine in its molecular structure—approximately 37.3% of its molecular weight. When metabolized in the liver, iodine is released and accumulates in hepatocytes. This accumulation increases liver density on CT scans and is considered a key factor in hepatotoxicity.

2.2 Mechanisms of hepatocyte injury

Although the exact mechanisms by which iodine accumulation causes hepatocyte injury are not fully understood, several pathways are believed to contribute to liver cell damage:

2.2.1 Oxidative stress

Iodine can act as an oxidizing agent, leading to the production of reactive oxygen species (ROS) within hepatocytes [5]. The excessive generation of ROS overwhelms the liver's antioxidant defenses, such as glutathione, resulting in oxidative stress. Oxidative stress damages cellular components—including lipids, proteins, and DNA—leading to hepatocyte apoptosis or necrosis. This cellular damage contributes to liver inflammation and can progress to fibrosis if the oxidative stress persists.

2.2.2 Phospholipidosis

Amiodarone induces phospholipidosis by causing the accumulation of phospholipids within hepatocytes [3]. The drug interferes with phospholipid metabolism, leading to the formation of intracellular lamellar bodies. This accumulation disrupts normal cellular functions by altering membrane fluidity and impairing organelle function. Excess phospholipids change the composition and fluidity of cellular membranes, affecting membrane-bound enzymes and receptors. The buildup in organelles like mitochondria and lysosomes hinders their function, leading to energy deficits and impaired detoxification processes. These disruptions lead to hepatocyte dysfunction and can initiate cell death pathways.

2.2.3 Immune-mediated injury

Some studies suggest that amiodarone or its metabolites may act as haptens, binding to liver proteins and forming neoantigens. This can trigger an immune response where the body's immune system mistakenly attacks its own hepatocytes [6]. The immune-mediated injury involves activation of cytotoxic T cells that target and destroy hepatocytes presenting the neoantigens. Additionally, the release of pro-inflammatory cytokines like tumor necrosis factor-alpha (TNF-α) and interleukins amplifies the inflammatory response. The formation of autoantibodies against liver tissues may further perpetuate the damage, leading to inflammation and potentially contributing to chronic liver conditions if not addressed promptly.

3. Clinical manifestations of amiodarone-induced hepatotoxicity

Amiodarone-induced hepatotoxicity presents a spectrum of clinical manifestations, ranging from asymptomatic elevations in liver enzymes to acute liver failure. Understanding these manifestations is crucial for early detection and management.

3.1 Asymptomatic elevations

Many patients undergoing amiodarone therapy exhibit elevated liver enzymes such as alanine aminotransferase (ALT) and aspartate aminotransferase (AST) without noticeable symptoms. These asymptomatic elevations are markers of hepatocyte injury and are often detected through routine blood tests. Regular monitoring of liver function tests is essential to identify hepatotoxicity at an early stage.

3.2 Nonspecific symptoms

Some patients may experience nonspecific symptoms that can be easily overlooked or attributed to other causes. These include fatigue, a general feeling of tiredness or weakness not relieved by rest; nausea, a sensation of stomach unease that may lead to an urge to vomit; abdominal discomfort, pain or discomfort in the upper right quadrant of the abdomen where the liver is located; and loss of appetite, a decreased desire to eat, potentially leading to unintended weight loss. These symptoms may indicate mild to moderate liver dysfunction and warrant further investigation.

3.3 Severe liver dysfunction

In rare instances, amiodarone-induced hepatotoxicity can progress to severe liver dysfunction, presenting with more serious clinical signs. These include jaundice, or yellowing of the skin and eyes due to elevated bilirubin levels, indicating significant liver impairment; coagulopathy, which is impaired blood clotting leading to easy bruising or excessive bleeding, as the liver produces essential clotting factors; hepatic encephalopathy, a decline in brain function resulting from the liver's inability to remove toxins from the blood, causing confusion, altered levels of consciousness, and even coma; ascites, the accumulation of fluid in the abdominal cavity due to decreased protein synthesis and increased pressure in the liver vessels; and pruritus, severe itching caused by bile salt accumulation in the skin.

4. Limitations of traditional diagnostic methods for amiodarone-induced hepatotoxicity

4.1 Limitations of liver function tests

Liver function tests (LFTs) are commonly used to monitor liver health in patients undergoing amiodarone therapy. These tests primarily measure levels of enzymes such as alanine aminotransferase (ALT) and aspartate aminotransferase (AST), which are indicators of hepatocellular injury. Despite their widespread use, LFTs have notable limitations. Elevated ALT and AST levels indicate liver cell damage but do not specify the underlying cause. Other conditions, including viral hepatitis, alcoholic liver disease, or the use of different hepatotoxic medications, can also result in elevated liver enzymes. This lack of specificity makes it challenging to attribute liver dysfunction solely to amiodarone. Additionally, LFTs do not provide information about the accumulation of iodine in the liver, a key factor in amiodarone-induced hepatotoxicity. Consequently, patients may exhibit normal liver enzyme levels despite having significant iodine deposition and underlying liver injury. Furthermore, LFTs may not detect early liver damage. By the time significant abnormalities in liver enzymes are observed, substantial hepatocellular injury may have already occurred. Early subtle changes in liver function can go unnoticed, delaying diagnosis and intervention.

4.2 Limitations of single-energy CT scans

Single-energy computed tomography (CT) scans are another traditional diagnostic tool used to evaluate liver alterations in patients taking amiodarone. However, these scans also present several limitations. Single-energy CT scans lack the capability to distinguish iodine accumulation from other substances like fat within the liver. In patients with concurrent hepatic steatosis, the presence of fat can obscure or mimic the increased liver density caused by iodine deposition, leading to potential false-negative results. Additionally, the accuracy of single-energy CT scans in assessing hepatic iodine concentration is affected by technical variables such as tube voltage settings and beam hardening artifacts. These factors can distort CT attenuation values, resulting in inaccurate measurements of liver density and iodine accumulation.

4.3 Summary of limitations

Traditional diagnostic methods for amiodarone-induced hepatotoxicity, including liver function tests and single-energy CT scans, exhibit significant limitations. These methods lack specificity, as they cannot specifically attribute liver injury to amiodarone or accurately quantify iodine accumulation within the liver. They are often ineffective in identifying early stages of liver injury, reducing the opportunity for timely medical intervention. Moreover, the inability to precisely measure hepatic iodine concentration hampers the assessment of the extent of iodine-induced liver damage. These limitations highlight the necessity for more advanced diagnostic tools that offer specific, early, and accurate evaluation of hepatic iodine accumulation and liver injury in patients undergoing long-term amiodarone therapy. Emerging imaging techniques and biomarkers may provide improved sensitivity and specificity, facilitating better management of amiodarone-induced hepatotoxicity.

5. Principles and advantages of dual-energy CT

Dual-energy computed tomography (DECT) is an advanced imaging technology that utilizes two different X-ray energy levels to acquire images, providing more detailed tissue information than traditional single-energy CT scans. This technology offers substantial clinical advantages, especially for evaluating hepatic iodine concentration induced by amiodarone therapy.

5.1 Principles of dual-energy CT

DECT employs two X-ray beams at distinct energy levels—typically 100 kVp (kilovolt peak) and 140 kVp—to scan the patient either simultaneously or sequentially. This dual-energy approach enhances tissue differentiation by exploiting the varying interactions of X-rays with different body tissues. For instance, higher-energy X-rays penetrate iodine more effectively, while lower-energy X-rays are more readily absorbed by iodine atoms. By analyzing the differences in attenuation between the two energy levels, DECT can accurately distinguish tissue types and quantify specific substances like iodine, using advanced algorithms to produce material-specific images for precise identification and quantification [7].

5.2 Advantages of DECT in evaluating amiodarone-induced hepatic iodine concentration

5.2.1 Accurate quantification of iodine concentration

DECT allows for precise quantification of iodine concentration in the liver, overcoming the limitations of traditional single-energy CT scans. This is particularly beneficial in distinguishing iodine from other substances, such as fat, which can affect CT attenuation values. This capability is essential for patients with hepatic steatosis, as DECT ensures accurate iodine concentration measurements without interference from fat.

5.2.2 Non-invasive diagnostic tool

As a non-invasive modality, DECT reduces the need for procedures like liver biopsies, thereby minimizing patient discomfort and associated risks. This tool is also valuable for monitoring the hepatotoxic side effects of amiodarone therapy, facilitating early clinical interventions when necessary.

5.2.3 Early detection of liver injury

DECT's ability to precisely measure hepatic iodine concentration enables earlier detection of liver injury compared to conventional methods. This allows for timely adjustments to the treatment regimen, such as modifying the dosage or discontinuing amiodarone, ultimately improving patient outcomes by preventing progression of liver injury.

5.2.4 Virtual non-contrast imaging (VNC)

DECT can generate virtual non-contrast (VNC) images by subtracting the iodine component from contrast-enhanced scans, simulating unenhanced CT images. This approach allows for a more accurate assessment of liver parenchyma, particularly in cases of iodine accumulation, and aids in detecting hepatic steatosis that might be obscured in traditional contrast-enhanced scans.

5.2.5 Monitoring changes in hepatic iodine concentration

DECT can also track changes in hepatic iodine concentration over time, enabling clinicians to evaluate the efficacy and safety of amiodarone therapy. This continuous monitoring supports personalized treatment plans tailored to each patient's specific therapeutic response.

5.3 Summary

In summary, DECT is a powerful imaging technology that provides several advantages in assessing amiodarone-induced hepatic iodine concentration. Key benefits include enhanced accuracy in quantifying iodine concentration, reduced need for invasive procedures, early detection capabilities, advanced imaging options such as Virtual Non-Contrast imaging, and the ability to monitor hepatic changes longitudinally, informing ongoing treatment decisions.

6. Scanning parameters, ROI selection, and measurement methods for liver iodine concentration using dual-energy CT (DECT)

Based on available data and previous discussions, the following recommended protocol for monitoring hepatic injury due to amiodarone uses the Siemens SOMATOM Definition Flash CT scanner as an example.

6.1 Scanning range

The scanning range should encompass the superior and inferior borders of the liver. The patient should raise both arms and hold their breath after exhaling during the scan.

6.2 Scanning parameters

Collimation is set to 32 × 0.6 mm. Rotation time is 0.5 seconds with a pitch of 0.6 and a slice thickness of 0.6 mm. Tube voltage includes Tube A at 100 kV and Tube B at Sn 140 kV, utilizing a tin filter for optimal spectral separation. Tube current for both Tube A and Tube B uses automatic mAs with automatic exposure control, incorporating CARE Dose4D technology to optimize radiation dose and ensure patient safety.

6.3 Image reconstruction

The reconstruction algorithm utilizes the D30f kernel for all images, with a reconstruction interval of 0.7 mm and a slice thickness of 1.5 mm.

6.4 Iodine concentration measurement

The Siemens syngo.via workstation (version VB20B) is used, with non-contrast DECT images imported into the Dual-Energy software. Selecting the "Liver Virtual Non-Contrast (VNC)" mode enables automatic energy subtraction and generates iodine distribution images. Regions of interest (ROIs) are drawn in liver segments II/III, IV, V/VI, and VII/VIII, each with an area of at least 1 cm^2. ROIs should avoid including vascular structures or bile ducts, and iodine concentration is recorded for each liver segment.

6.5 Follow-up monitoring

For patients on long-term amiodarone therapy, regular DECT scans are recommended to monitor hepatic iodine concentration changes. During follow-ups, scanning a single slice at the largest cross-sectional area of the liver is advised to reduce radiation exposure while ensuring accurate assessments. The frequency of follow-up scans should be tailored to individual risk factors such as amiodarone dosage, therapy duration, baseline liver function, and any existing liver conditions, with high-risk patients requiring more frequent monitoring and low-risk patients having extended intervals.

6.6 Additional recommendations

DECT results should be interpreted alongside clinical presentation, liver function tests, and findings from other imaging modalities. A multidisciplinary approach is essential for an accurate liver status assessment. If amiodarone-induced liver injury is suspected, adjust treatment promptly by reducing dosage, discontinuing amiodarone, or considering alternative therapies. Close monitoring of liver function tests is necessary to prevent the progression of hepatic damage.

6.7 Important considerations

Customized protocols are advised, as the recommended parameters are based on specific research and may not universally apply. Scanning protocols should be adjusted based on patient needs, equipment capabilities, and clinical requirements, with consultation from radiology experts for personalized guidance. Adherence to the ALARA principle is crucial for radiation safety, minimizing exposure by limiting follow-up scans to a single slice to balance imaging benefits with radiation risks. Ensure ethical and legal compliance with institutional policies and relevant regulations, obtaining informed patient consent where appropriate, especially when modifying standard protocols.

Note: This protocol serves as a general guideline. Tailoring the scanning protocol to each patient's condition is essential, and consulting experienced professionals when designing imaging strategies is recommended.

7. Correlation between DECT-measured hepatic iodine concentration and liver function impairment

Studies have demonstrated a significant correlation between hepatic iodine concentration measured by dual-energy CT (DECT) and the degree of liver function impairment in patients undergoing amiodarone therapy.

7.1 Significance of DECT-measured iodine concentration

DECT provides an accurate, non-invasive method to quantify hepatic iodine accumulation associated with amiodarone use. Elevated hepatic iodine concentrations detected by DECT have been linked to hepatocellular injury, as indicated by abnormalities in liver function tests.

7.2 Clinical findings

7.2.1 Positive correlation with liver enzymes

Patients with higher hepatic iodine concentrations measured by DECT often exhibit elevated liver enzyme levels, such as alanine aminotransferase (ALT) and aspartate aminotransferase (AST). This correlation suggests that DECT-measured iodine concentration can serve as a surrogate marker for amiodarone-induced hepatotoxicity.

7.2.2 Threshold levels and risk assessment

To assess the risk of liver function impairment, it is essential to calculate the hepatic amiodarone concentration and compare it against established safety thresholds. The iodine content in amiodarone's molecular structure is approximately 37.3% by mass [8]. The concentration of amiodarone ($C_{\text{amiodarone}}$) can be calculated using the formula:

$$C_{\text{amiodarone}} = \frac{\text{Ciodine}}{0.373} \quad (1)$$

where $C_{amiodarone}$ represents the concentration of amiodarone (mg/mL) and C_{iodine} is the measured iodine concentration (mg/mL).

Safety thresholds: According to research, when serum amiodarone concentration exceeds 2.5 mg/L, the risk of liver function impairment increases. Since hepatic amiodarone concentration is typically about 500 times the serum concentration, the liver concentration should remain below 1250 mg/L (1.25 mg/mL). This corresponds to a hepatic iodine concentration upper limit of:

$$C_{iodine}, safe = 1.25 mg / mL \times 0.373 = 0.4663 mg / mL \qquad (2)$$

Safety range for hepatic amiodarone concentration: The safety threshold for hepatic amiodarone concentration is 1.25 mg/mL (based on findings that serum amiodarone concentrations greater than 2.5 mg/L may cause liver function damage, and hepatic amiodarone concentrations are approximately 500 times the serum levels).

Since 1.073 mg/mL < 1.25 mg/mL, the hepatic amiodarone concentration is within the safe range.

Safety range for hepatic iodine concentration: Calculation of the corresponding hepatic iodine safety threshold:

Therefore, the hepatic iodine concentration must remain below 0.4663 mg/mL.

Determining iodine concentration safety: Since 0.4 mg/mL < 0.4663 mg/mL, the hepatic iodine concentration is also within the safe range.

In clinical practice, the measured hepatic iodine concentration should be compared to this safety threshold of 0.466 mg/mL to guide potential adjustments in amiodarone dosing, reducing the risk of adverse reactions due to drug accumulation.

7.3 Clinical implications

7.3.1 Early detection and intervention

By detecting elevated hepatic iodine levels before significant liver damage occurs, clinicians can adjust amiodarone dosage or consider alternative treatments. Early intervention may prevent progression to severe hepatotoxicity, improving patient outcomes.

7.3.2 Personalized patient management

Patients with higher hepatic iodine concentrations may require more frequent liver function monitoring and follow-up imaging studies. Quantitative data from DECT aids in making evidence-based decisions regarding the continuation or modification of amiodarone therapy.

7.4 Limitations and future directions

Existing studies on DECT-measured hepatic iodine concentration and liver function impairment often involve small patient populations, which limits the robustness of the correlation. Additionally, variations in DECT scanning protocols and measurement techniques can impact the consistency and comparability of results. Future research should focus on conducting large-scale, multicenter studies to validate this correlation. Standardizing DECT protocols and establishing consensus on threshold values are crucial for broader clinical adoption. Furthermore, integrating DECT findings with other diagnostic markers could enhance the accuracy of hepatotoxicity assest.

8. Clinical casmense presentation

8.1 Case study: Amiodarone-induced hepatotoxicity detected by DECT

8.1.1 Medical history and laboratory findings

A 66-year-old male patient with atrial fibrillation, maintained on oral amiodarone at 200 mg/day for 10 years, showed elevated liver enzyme levels in routine laboratory evaluations: alanine aminotransferase (ALT) at 127 IU/L (reference range: 9–50 IU/L), aspartate aminotransferase (AST) at 101 IU/L (reference range: 15–40 IU/L), and gamma-glutamyl transferase (GGT) at 1080 IU/L (reference range: 120–250 IU/L). These findings indicate hepatocellular injury and potential cholestasis (**Figures 1–3**).

8.1.2 Summary

The patient was diagnosed with amiodarone-induced hepatotoxicity based on elevated liver enzymes and DECT findings of increased hepatic iodine concentration. Following diagnosis, amiodarone therapy was discontinued, and the patient subsequently underwent radiofrequency ablation for atrial fibrillation management. This case highlights the effectiveness of DECT in detecting hepatic iodine accumulation, enabling early diagnosis and intervention to prevent further liver damage.

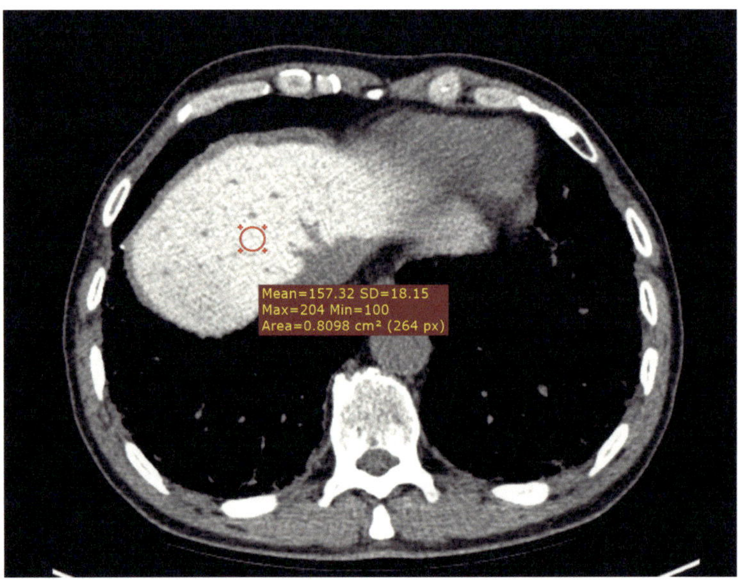

Figure 1.
Axial CT image at 100 kV showing hepatic segment VIII with a region of interest (ROI) measuring a CT attenuation value of 157 Hounsfield Units (HU).

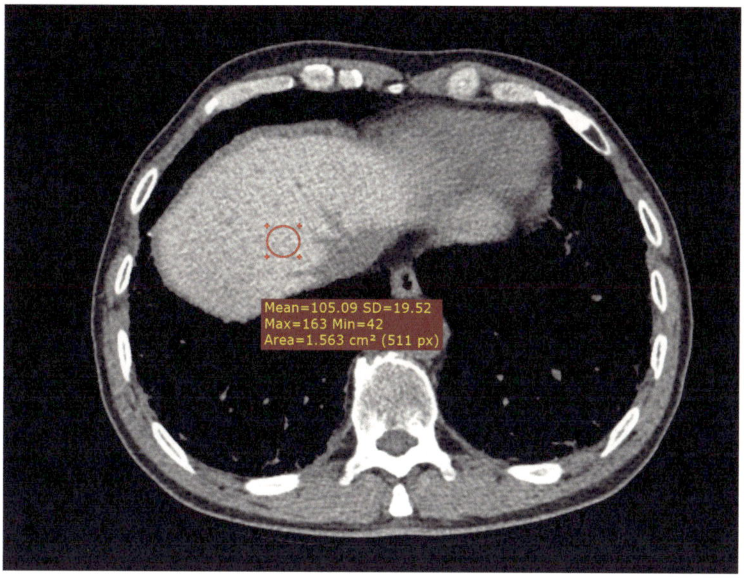

Figure 2.
Axial CT image at 140 kV showing the same ROI in hepatic segment VIII with a CT attenuation value of 105 HU.

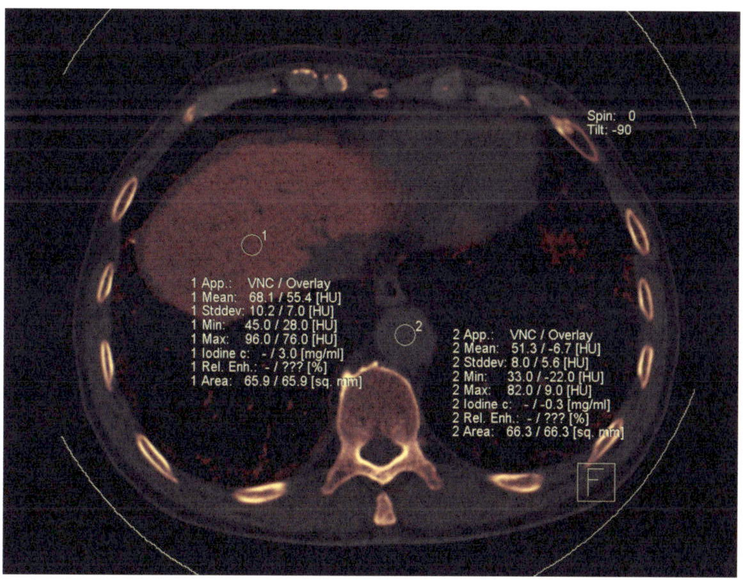

Figure 3.
Dual-energy CT (DECT) iodine map illustrating hepatic iodine concentration of 3.0 mg/mL in hepatic segment VIII (ROI 1) and a virtual non-contrast (VNC) liver CT value of 68 HU.

9. Conclusions

Non-contrast DECT is emerging as a quantitative and non-invasive approach for measuring hepatic iodine concentration, offering a feasible and novel biomarker for monitoring amiodarone-induced hepatotoxicity. By integrating DECT measurements with liver function tests, clinicians can achieve early diagnosis of amiodarone-induced liver injury, thereby preventing progression to irreversible stages, such as cirrhosis.

Studies indicate that timely discontinuation of amiodarone can lead to normalization of both elevated liver CT density and abnormal liver function tests [9], suggesting that amiodarone accumulation in the liver may be a reversible dynamic process. This reversibility underscores the importance of early detection and intervention, as prompt cessation of the drug can restore normal liver function and structure.

Additionally, DECT can aid in differentiating increased liver density due to conditions like hemochromatosis and hemosiderosis, thus improving diagnostic accuracy and ensuring appropriate treatment strategies. DECT's capability to distinguish between various causes of elevated liver density enhances its clinical value, especially in settings where differential diagnosis is essential.

Looking forward, advancements such as three-dimensional (3D) DECT measurement techniques could enable precise quantification of total hepatic iodine content, offering further clinical benefit to patients on long-term oral amiodarone therapy. Such quantification would facilitate comprehensive assessments of hepatic iodine distribution and accumulation, allowing for more personalized treatment plans that optimize therapeutic efficacy while minimizing hepatotoxicity risk.

Incorporating DECT into routine clinical practice represents a significant step forward in the non-invasive evaluation of drug-induced liver injury. Should multicenter, large-scale studies corroborate these findings, DECT could be integrated into clinical guidelines and standard protocols for monitoring amiodarone-induced hepatotoxicity. Such standardization would improve early detection rates, enhance patient outcomes, and ultimately standardize patient care.

In summary, DECT is a promising tool for clinicians to accurately and non-invasively monitor hepatic iodine accumulation. Its application enables early diagnosis, improved risk stratification, and informed decision-making in managing patients on long-term amiodarone therapy. Embracing DECT technology aligns with precision medicine, where tailored interventions based on individual data enhance healthcare delivery and patient well-being.

10. Main findings

1. *Correlation between hepatic iodine concentration and liver enzyme levels*: DECT measurements reveal that patients on long-term amiodarone therapy have significantly elevated hepatic iodine concentrations. This iodine increase correlates positively with liver enzyme markers, particularly ALT and AST, indicating a direct association between iodine accumulation and hepatocellular injury.

2. *Threshold for hepatotoxicity*: The analysis identifies a hepatic iodine concentration threshold of 0.47 mg/mL, beyond which the risk of liver function impairment markedly increases. Approximately 6% of patients exceeding this iodine threshold developed abnormal liver function.

3. *Comparative diagnostic value of DECT*: Compared to traditional single-energy CT scans, DECT provides superior accuracy in quantifying iodine concentration without interference from confounding factors like hepatic steatosis. DECT effectively distinguishes iodine accumulation from fat deposits, improving the identification of hepatic injury extent in patients on amiodarone therapy.

Conflict of interest

The authors declare no conflict of interest.

Author details

Hongwei Zhao*, Hu Liu and Haijuan Lv
Department of Radiology, Second Affiliated Hospital of Jiaxing University, Jiaxing, Zhejiang Province, China

*Address all correspondence to: zhw0314@hotmail.com

References

[1] Vassallo P, Trohman RG. Prescribing amiodarone: An evidence-based review of clinical indications. JAMA. 2007;**298**(11):1312-1322. DOI: 10.1001/jama.298.11.1312

[2] Gayam V, Khalid M, Dahal S, et al. Fatal acute liver failure with intravenous amiodarone: A case report and literature review. Gastroenterology Research. 2018;**11**(1):62-63. DOI: 10.14740/gr911w

[3] Goldman IS, Winkler ML, Raper SE, et al. Increased hepatic density and phospholipidosis due to amiodarone. AJR. American Journal of Roentgenology. 1985;**144**(3):541-546. DOI: 10.2214/ajr.144.3.541

[4] Lv HJ, Zhao HW. Amiodarone-induced hepatotoxicity - quantitative measurement of iodine density in the liver using dual-energy computed tomography: Three case reports. World Journal of Clinical Cases. 2020;**8**(20):4958-4965. DOI: 10.12998/wjcc.v8.i20.4958

[5] Takai S, Oda S, Tsuneyama K, et al. Establishment of a mouse model for amiodarone-induced liver injury and analyses of its hepatotoxic mechanism. Journal of Applied Toxicology. 2016;**36**(1):35-47. DOI: 10.1002/jat.3141

[6] Nacca N, Bhamidipati CM, Yuhico LS, et al. Severe amiodarone induced pulmonary toxicity. Journal of Thoracic Disease. 2012;**4**(6):667-670. DOI: 10.3978/j.issn.2072-1439.2012.06.08

[7] Koonce JD, Vliegenthart R, Schoepf UJ, et al. Accuracy of dual-energy computed tomography for the measurement of iodine concentration using cardiac CT protocols: Validation in a phantom model. European Radiology. 2014;**24**(2):512-518. DOI: 10.1007/s00330-013-3040-6

[8] Trohman RG, Sharma PS, Mcaninch EA, et al. Amiodarone and thyroid physiology, pathophysiology, diagnosis and management. Trends in Cardiovascular Medicine. 2019;**29**(5):285-295. DOI: 10.1016/j.tcm.2018.09.005

[9] Kojima S, Kojima S, Ueno H, et al. Increased density of the liver and amiodarone-associated phospholipidosis. Cardiology Research and Practice. 2009;**2009**:598940. DOI: 10.4061/2009/598940

Section 2

Hepatotoxicity in Other Aspects

Chapter 5

Metabolic Hepatic Alterations and Disease under Hypoxic Conditions

Eduardo Pena and Marco Luza

Abstract

Hypoxia refers to a decrease in oxygen levels in cells, tissues, organs and organisms. This condition can be generated by several factors, where a series of acclimatization processes lead to the generation of different responses at the physiological and molecular levels in aerobic living beings to compensate for the decrease in oxygen. One of the alterations in this condition is an increase in triglyceride and total cholesterol concentrations, which is related to metabolic pathway alterations, resulting in an increase in the gene expression of sterol regulatory element-binding proteins (SREBPs) in the liver, which in some cases could trigger nonalcoholic hepatic steatosis pathology in aerobic organisms. From research on hypoxemic hypoxia, this scientific chapter compiles information on the influence of hypobaric and normobaric hypoxia on physiological and metabolic alterations at the hepatic level, as well as its possible implications for the subsequent development of hepatic diseases. In conclusion, hypoxic conditions are directly related to alterations in the metabolic pathways of lipids and cholesterol mediated by SREBPs, altering the expression of stearoyl-CoA desaturase-1 (SCD-1), transcription factor peroxisome proliferator-activated receptor gamma (PPAR-γ) and 3-hydroxy-3-methyl-glutaryl-CoA reductase (HMG-CoA) at the hepatic level and increasing the concentrations of triglycerides and cholesterol in the liver.

Keywords: hypobaric hypoxia, normobaric hypoxia, metabolic alterations, liver, SREBP, hypertriglyceridemia, hypercholesterolemia

1. Introduction

Hypoxia is characterized by a decrease in oxygen bioavailability in cells, tissues, organs and organisms. This condition can be generated by several factors that induce different kinds of hypoxia, such as anemia, stagnation, cytotoxicity and hypoxemic hypoxia, where a series of acclimatization processes and physiological responses are necessary to compensate for the hypoxic conditions. Under high-altitude conditions, the partial pressure of oxygen decreases due to the decrease in barometric pressure in the atmosphere. This effect is known as hypobaric hypoxia, which is characterized by a reduction in the oxygen tension at the level of the pulmonary alveolus, cells, and tissues. This deficiency in oxygen bioavailability leads to alterations in metabolic pathways and the functions of various organs in aerobic organisms [1].

In Chile, approximately 80,000 people live and work under high-altitude conditions (2500 m above sea level), where owing to mining activities, the number of people exposed to these conditions has been increasing in the northern regions of the country [2]. In this context, a significant percentage of the workforce is subjected to high-altitude work activities through rotating shifts alternating between work at high altitude and rest at sea level for years, which has been defined as a model of chronic intermittent hypobaric hypoxia exposure [3]. Studies have shown that this condition causes a series of physiological alterations in individuals, leading to pathologies such as acute mountain sickness (AMS), high-altitude pulmonary edema (HAPE), high-altitude pulmonary hypertension (HAPH) and high-altitude cerebral edema (HACE), which are described below.

On the other hand, from a metabolic perspective, studies have shown that hypobaric hypoxia induces anorexia, increased lipolysis, and an elevated metabolic rate, among other effects [2, 4, 5]. In the last 50 years, obesity in individuals, defined as excessive or abnormal accumulation of fat (BMI > 30), which is detrimental to health, has become a global issue. According to studies by the World Health Organization (WHO) and the Organization for Economic Cooperation and Development (OECD), approximately 40% of the population is overweight [6]. In Chile, in 2016, 74% of the population was obese, and particularly, the Tarapacá Region had an obesity rate of 31.46%, which is notable considering the number of people who live and work in these conditions [2].

There are different types of hypobaric hypoxia depending on the duration of exposure; for example, acute hypobaric hypoxia, such as AMS, also known as soroche or puna, which includes symptoms such as dizziness, nausea, vomiting, loss of consciousness, memory loss, headaches, and dyspnea. These symptoms are rapidly reversed with exposure to oxygen at sea level. Additionally, under these conditions, HAPE and HACE, which can lead to death, develop. On the other hand, chronic hypobaric hypoxia, such as chronic mountain sickness (CMS), excessive erythrocytosis, Monge's disease, and HAPH, results in persistent alterations over time [7, 8]. According to León-Velarde and colleagues, intermittent chronic hypobaric hypoxia may present characteristics of both previously mentioned conditions [9].

Studies have shown that this hypoxic condition is also associated with alterations in lipid biosynthesis [5]. Importantly, exposure to hypoxia results in the stabilization of transcription factors, such as hypoxia-inducible factor (HIF) [5, 10, 11]. Hypoxia-inducible factors (HIFs) act as transcription factors that regulate various physiological and pathological processes by the overexpression of target genes [12].

On the other hand, there is another normobaric hypoxic condition, specifically, chronic intermittent normobaric hypoxia, induced by obstructive sleep apnea (OSA), which presents in some alterations observed in hypobaric hypoxia, indicating that some similar molecular pathways exist between both hypoxic conditions [11, 13]. However, it is important to note that both hypoxia conditions could also differ in terms of metabolic pathways at the molecular level. Therefore, in this study, they were contrasted to better determine the possible pathways that affect lipid synthesis. Therefore, the objective of this study was to determine the alterations in specific proteins involved in hepatic metabolism under different conditions of hypobaric and normobaric hypoxia.

2. Types of hypoxia

Hypoxia is a condition characterized by a reduction in the bioavailability of O_2, which leads to a decrease in this vital gas at the level of organs, tissues, cells, and cellular organelles in aerobic organisms [14].

There are several types of hypoxia, such as anemic hypoxia, which is related to a decrease in the oxygen-carrying capacity of the blood; stagnation hypoxia, which is related to a decrease in blood flow; cytotoxic hypoxia, caused by the use of drugs or medications; and hypoxemic hypoxia, which is caused by a decrease in oxygen in the blood [15]. Hypoxemic hypoxia can be divided into two subgroups: normobaric hypoxia and hypobaric hypoxia [15].

Normobaric hypoxia occurs due to the inhalation of air with low concentrations of oxygen (>20%), which is generally observed in patients with obstructive sleep apnea (OSA) [15]. The second group corresponds to hypobaric hypoxia, a condition caused by a decrease in atmospheric pressure, where the partial pressure of oxygen also decreases, leading to reduced gas exchange at the pulmonary alveolar level and subsequently in the venous blood of the pulmonary capillaries, resulting in hypoxemia at the organism level [3]. In this study, we focused on hypoxemic hypoxia.

3. Types of hypobaric hypoxia

There are several classifications of hypobaric hypoxia, depending on the duration of exposure to high-altitude conditions (geographic altitudes above 2500 m above sea level). We begin by defining the model of acute hypobaric hypoxia, which is characterized by a short period, primarily between hours or days [3]. The chronic hypobaric hypoxia model is characterized by prolonged exposure (in years) under high-altitude conditions and is primarily observed in natives of the Andes, Himalayas, and Sherpas [16–19]. Recent studies have highlighted their genetic adaptability to high-altitude exposure [16].

In recent years, many Chilean mining models operate at high altitudes by rotating shifts, with the most common being a 7-day work shift at high altitude followed by 7 days of rest at sea level, creating an alternating pattern between high-altitude and sea-level conditions, known in biomedical terms as intermittent chronic hypobaric hypoxia [3]. On the other hand, a decrease in the partial pressure of oxygen or hypobaric hypoxia can trigger a series of genetic responses and, subsequently, protein-level responses [20]. This can lead to alterations in physiology, specifically focusing on hepatic levels, which will be presented and discussed below.

4. Effect of hypobaric hypoxia on hepatic metabolism

The liver plays a crucial role in controlling lipid homeostasis through various activities, including the synthesis, oxidation, metabolism, storage, and distribution of lipids. Triglycerides, the main lipid molecules, serve as a source of fatty acids in liver tissue [12]. When our body needs energy (ATP), fatty acids are broken down through β-oxidation to produce acetyl-CoA, which then enters the citric acid cycle and subsequently undergoes oxidative phosphorylation. If energy levels in the body are sufficient, fatty acids are stored as triglycerides in the liver. However, under hypobaric hypoxic conditions, this metabolic pathway is inhibited, leading to the synthesis of fatty acids into triglycerides within hepatocytes [12, 21].

Hypoxia-inducible factor (HIF) is a molecule with different subunits; the HIF-α subunit is sensitive to oxygen deprivation, whereas the HIF-β subunit is a constitutive molecule that stabilizes the HIF molecule [12]. As previously mentioned, HIF is a transcription factor expressed in all organisms and plays an essential role in maintaining oxygen homeostasis [22]. Under hypoxic conditions, HIF-1 regulates the transcription of hundreds of genes in a cell-specific manner, with the HIF-1α isoform involved in physiological and developmental pathways that supply O_2 to cells or enable cells to survive under conditions of reduced oxygen bioavailability [22]. For example, HIF-1 is related to several physiological processes under hypoxic conditions, such as angiogenesis, invasion, metabolic reprogramming, hypoxic pulmonary vasoconstriction, and vascular and cardiac remodeling [23, 24].

In addition, HIF has been described as related to alterations in the pathways of cholesterol and triglyceride biosynthesis, leading to increased lipid levels in liver tissue and plasma, which can cause liver damage [5]. Studies by Siques and collaborators concluded that chronic exposure to hypobaric hypoxia similarly affects lipid levels in plasma and the liver, highlighting an increase in triglyceride and very low-density lipoprotein (vLDL) cholesterol levels, primarily mediated by the upregulation of stearoyl-CoA desaturase-1 (SCD-1), a key enzyme in lipid metabolism that catalyzes the desaturation of saturated fatty acids, specifically the conversion of stearic acid into oleic acid, which is a monounsaturated fatty acid. SCD-1 is involved in regulating the balance between saturated and unsaturated fatty acids in cell membranes and adipose tissue. Its function has a direct effect on lipid synthesis and metabolic processes such as lipogenesis, the regulation of insulin resistance and fat storage [25, 26]. These findings also emphasize the need for further research to explore other mechanisms that may contribute to these lipid alterations [5].

On the basis of these findings, studies conducted on animal models (Wistar rats) exposed to chronic hypobaric hypoxia (15 males at 4600 m above sea level for 30 days) also suggest alterations in the sterol regulatory element-binding protein (SREBP) [5], a family of transcription factors that play crucial roles in regulating lipid synthesis, particularly in the regulation of cholesterol and fatty acid metabolism [27]. SREBPs are proteins that, under conditions of lipid deficiency, are activated to increase the expression of genes involved in lipid biosynthesis. There are different isoforms, SREBP-1, which is found mainly in the liver and is involved in fatty acid synthesis, and SREBP-2, which is crucial for regulating cholesterol metabolism by controlling genes that regulate cholesterol synthesis and uptake. SREBPs are synthesized as inactive precursors located in the endoplasmic reticulum [28]. Under conditions of lipid scarcity (such as cholesterol or fatty acids), SREBPs are transported through the Golgi apparatus, where they are processed by proteases to release the active form of the transcription factor, which then migrates to the nucleus to activate the expression of genes regulating lipid biosynthesis [29]. This, combined with increased triglyceride synthesis, results in elevated lipid levels in liver tissue and plasma, potentially leading to liver damage [5, 30]. On the other hand, studies on Sprague-Dawley rats exposed to chronic hypobaric hypoxia (12 males at 6700 m above sea level for 14 days) revealed an increase in taurine levels in urine [30], which is considered a biomarker for hepatic alterations [25]. Thus, exposure to chronic hypobaric hypoxia results in increased synthesis of triglycerides and cholesterol in hepatic cells.

With respect to intermittent hypobaric hypoxia conditions, studies on Wistar rats subjected to this type of hypobaric hypoxia (25 males at 7600 m above sea level for 5 minutes/week) revealed an increase in triacylglycerol levels in liver tissue, associated with the activation of acylglycerol-3-phosphate acyltransferase 2 and lipin-1—enzymes involved in triacylglycerol synthesis. Both are induced by the transcription factor peroxisome proliferator-activated receptor gamma (PPAR-γ), which is also regulated by HIF-1. Additionally, the same study showed that exposure to intermittent hypobaric hypoxia for more than a month does not increase the expression of HIF-1α mRNA, suggesting that mice exposed to prolonged intermittent hypobaric hypoxia may have undergone acclimatization. However, the results indicate that hepatic triacylglycerol synthesis under this type of hypobaric hypoxia could be regulated by the PPAR-γ transcription factor through HIF-1 stabilization. Therefore, increased early-stage expression of HIF-1α and PPAR-γ mRNAs during hypobaric hypoxia exposure would act as transcription factors to promote triacylglycerol synthesis in the liver [12].

Additionally, studies on Swiss albino mice under acute hypobaric hypoxia (10 males at 4600 m above sea level for 5 hours) suggest that liver tissue undergoes transcriptional changes in key genes involved in sterol and cholesterol metabolism, such as SREBP-1 and SREBP-2, respectively [31]. Importantly, physiological and pathological responses to different hypoxic conditions can vary both within and between species [32–34]. Therefore, both intermittent and chronic hypobaric hypoxia exposure generate hepatic alterations through increased triglycerides and cholesterol, involving proteins such as HIF, PPAR-γ, SCD-1, HMG-CoA reductase, SREBP-1, and SREBP-2 in the liver, whereas exposure to SREBP-1 and 2 is associated with increased sterol and cholesterol levels.

To our knowledge, there is limited information on the condition of hypobaric hypoxia and its effect on hepatic metabolism. This led us to study normobaric hypoxia, with the aim of enhancing the understanding of the protein alterations involved in hepatic metabolic pathways under hypoxic conditions, which will be explained below.

5. Effects of normobaric hypoxia on hepatic metabolism

Like what is observed in hypobaric hypoxia conditions, normobaric hypoxia affects hepatic metabolism. These effects are not directly associated with an increase in dietary intake but rather with exposure to hypoxia itself. Studies have demonstrated that the concentrations of triglycerides and diacylglycerides increase significantly under normobaric hypoxic conditions. It is proposed that this condition indirectly affects specific lipids and fatty acids by altering their absorption. Additionally, normobaric hypoxia can directly modify metabolic pathways in the liver, leading to conditions such as nonalcoholic fatty liver disease (NAFLD) [35].

Studies in neonatal Sprague-Dawley mice have shown that under normobaric hypoxic conditions (12% O_2; 7 days, 60 pups, mixed sex), there is an increase in triglycerides in the blood, brain, and liver [14]. In the liver, it has been proposed that this increase is due to elevated de novo synthesis, a process by which circulating carbohydrates are converted into fatty acids [35]. *De novo* synthesis primarily occurs in adipose tissue, but under normobaric hypoxic conditions, this synthesis is reduced in adipose tissue and increased in hepatic tissue, potentially contributing to pathological liver development, such as NAFLD [14]. Importantly, acute normobaric hypoxia conditions have been shown to alter cholesterol levels in the liver, suggesting that this condition may induce metabolic imbalance in the body [35].

This study also revealed that the increase in the serum triglyceride concentration due to this condition is related to the inhibition of hepatic lipase, an enzyme similar to lipoprotein lipase (LPL), leading to impaired lipolysis in the bloodstream [14]. Additionally, the findings of this study suggest that this condition may also affect LPL activity [14], which could help elucidate the increased triglyceride release in the liver under chronic normobaric hypoxia exposure.

On the other hand, studies in C57BL/6 J mice, which are susceptible to diet-induced obesity, type 2 diabetes, and atherosclerosis, under intermittent chronic normobaric hypoxia conditions (5% O_2, 60 times per hour, 12 weeks, 40 males) have studied two groups: one with a cholesterol-rich diet and another with a regular diet. The results revealed the development of hyperlipidemia in both groups, regardless of baseline total cholesterol and LDL levels [13]. Additionally, this condition was found to elevate total serum cholesterol levels in both groups, which was associated with a significant increase in the hepatic levels of SCD-1 mRNA and protein [12]. Finally, this study revealed that cholesterol-rich diet-fed mice exposed to intermittent chronic normobaric hypoxia presented increased levels of proinflammatory cytokines in the liver, and this inflammatory process could be related to the development of atherosclerosis—the accumulation of fats, cholesterol, and other substances in the vascular wall, causing narrowing of hepatic arteries and blockage of blood flow in the liver [13].

As previously mentioned, HIF-1α plays a key role in biological processes under hypoxia, regulating the increase in glucose transporter transcription. Studies have proposed that exposure to normobaric hypoxia could be beneficial as a treatment for obesity and NAFLD since acclimatization to normobaric hypoxia results in the overexpression of genes regulating glycolysis. Current studies by Luo and colleagues in C57BL/6 mice under chronic intermittent normobaric hypoxia (10% O_2 for 1 hour/day, 16 males) suggest that it could be a noninvasive alternative to treat obesity and NAFLD, as their experiments revealed that it countered weight gain produced by a high-fat diet. Moreover, it reversed the increase in white and brown adipocytes and high-fat diet-induced fatty liver and protected liver function while regulating the expression of genes necessary for lipolysis, such as PPAR-γ, which was altered by the high-fat diet [36].

However, determining whether intermittent normobaric hypoxia exposure is a good treatment for NAFLD is questionable, since several studies focused on the same hypoxic conditions in C57BL/6 J mice have reported that HIF-1α stabilization might contribute to the development and exacerbation of NAFLD [10, 11, 30, 37–39]. In addition, it is important to highlight that in this study [36], the experimental procedure involved the use of 10% oxygen for 1 hour/day for this type of mouse, whereas in other studies that induced OSA (approximately 12 h of hypoxia) [10, 30, 37–39], the duration of hypoxia in this study was low (1 h), which only induced an increase in the epinephrine level, activating the physiological catabolism process; therefore, the underlying reason might be attributable to the use of different methods with a low intermittent dose of hypoxia. Therefore, further studies are needed to elucidate how the dose of hypoxia/reoxygenation in different animal models can affect liver tissue.

As previously mentioned, intermittent hypobaric hypoxia exposure induces HIF-1 transcriptional activity, suggesting that it can regulate SREBP-1 pathways and increase lipid biosynthesis [5]. This was also observed and corroborated by studies conducted on mice under chronic intermittent normobaric hypoxia (4.9% O_2/60 times per hour; 5 days), which documented a relationship between HIF-1α, triglyceride biosynthesis, overexpression of SCAP (SREBP cleavage-activating protein), SCD-1, and SREBP-1 levels. The activity of these proteins increases lipid biosynthesis in the liver. Previous studies have demonstrated that the overexpression of SREBP-1 and downstream lipid biosynthesis pathways, especially SCD-1, which controls the synthesis of monounsaturated fatty acids used as substrates for subsequent triglyceride biosynthesis, supports these findings [25, 40]. The role of HIF in this process is crucial, as a study in rodents with partial HIF-1α deficiency attenuated the increase in fasting serum and hepatic triglycerides, suggesting that normobaric hypoxia-induced hyperlipidemia could be directly mediated by HIF-1 [10, 11].

Importantly, SCD-1 is a key gene involved in the synthesis of monounsaturated fatty acids, which are the main substrates for triglyceride and hepatic phospholipid synthesis. Li and Grigoryev reported that SCD-1 is regulated by both SREBP-1 and exposure to intermittent chronic normobaric hypoxia (4.9% O_2; 5 days, 12 males). The overexpression of SCD-1 in response to intermittent hypoxia could explain the increases in triglyceride and phospholipid contents in the liver, leading to the progression of NAFLD [30]. Furthermore, this study also revealed that intermittent chronic hypoxia exacerbates preexisting fatty liver disease in genetically obese mice [30].

On the basis of these findings, studies in obese mice with obstructive sleep apnea or chronic intermittent normobaric hypoxia revealed that this condition, combined with obesity, results in increased expression of SREBPs, stimulating lipid biosynthesis in the liver [30].

On the other hand, studies agree that exposure to chronic intermittent normobaric hypoxia causes an increase in the hepatic expression of essential genes involved in regulating metabolic processes, mainly genes involved in lipid metabolism, such as SREBP-1, SREBP-2, HMG-CoA reductase, malic enzyme, acetyl-CoA synthetase, acetyl-CoA carboxylase, SCD-1, SCD-2, and the mitochondrial GPAT pathway. These findings suggest that chronic intermittent hypoxia is related to the upregulation

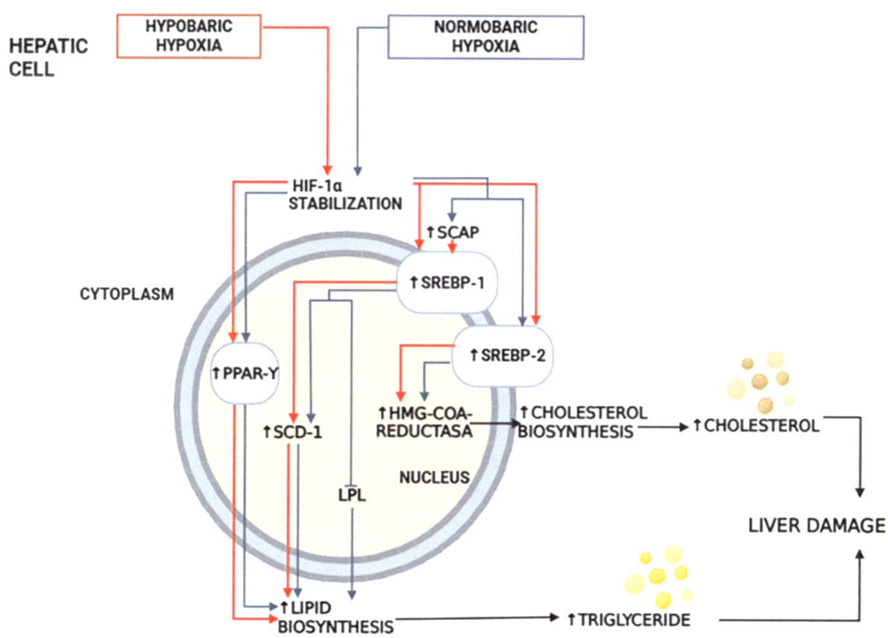

Figure 1.
Molecular signaling pathways involved in the alteration of lipid biosynthesis at the hepatic level in the development of liver damage induced by hypobaric and normobaric hypoxia conditions. Red represents molecular pathways under hypobaric hypoxia conditions, and blue represents molecular pathways under normobaric hypoxia conditions; PPAR-γ: peroxisome proliferator-activated receptor gamma; SREBP-1: sterol regulatory element-binding protein 1; SREBP-2: sterol regulatory element-binding protein 2; SCD-1: stearoyl-CoA desaturase-1; HMG-CoA reductase: 3-hydroxy-3-methyl-glutaryl-CoA reductase; LPL: lipoprotein lipase; SCAP: SREBP cleavage-activating protein.

of lipid biosynthesis pathways in the liver and increased levels of triglycerides and cholesterol, potentially exacerbating preexisting diseases and contributing to the development of NAFLD [30, 38, 41].

This finding is supported by subsequent studies in wild-type (WT) Hif1a+/+ and heterozygous-null (HET) Hif1a+/− mice with partial HIF-1α deficiency exposed to normobaric hypoxic conditions, which revealed a significant increase in the expression of key genes involved in fatty acid and triglyceride biosynthesis, such as SCAP, SREBP-1, and SCD-1, in WT mice. Specifically, SREBP-1 mRNA levels are higher in WT mice than in HET mice, whereas SREBP-2, the master regulator of cholesterol biosynthesis, is unaffected in both animal models [10, 11].

It is believed that HIF-1α affects SREBP-1 posttranscriptionally through SCAP, which facilitates the transport of SREBPs. This is because the SCAP gene promoter contains a putative binding site for HIF-1, suggesting that HIF-1 may upregulate liver lipid biosynthesis during normobaric hypoxia by stimulating SREBP-1 activity through SCAP [10, 11]. These findings suggest that lipid biosynthesis under normobaric hypoxic conditions is mediated by SREBP-1, SCD-1, and SCAP, with HIF playing a fundamental role in the development of NAFLD.

Figure 1 illustrates possible signaling pathways involved in alterations in hepatic lipid metabolism induced by exposure to hypobaric and normobaric hypoxia.

6. Hepatic metabolism under normobaric and hypobaric hypoxia

Based on the information presented above, both hypobaric and normobaric hypoxic conditions affect hepatic triglyceride and cholesterol biosynthesis, leading to hyperlipidemia and hypercholesterolemia. These conditions can cause hepatic imbalance, contributing to preexisting metabolic syndromes and the development of new chronic pathologies [10, 11, 30, 38, 39, 41]. Furthermore, in both hypobaric and normobaric hypoxia, exposure to high altitude stabilizes HIF-1α, which leads to the expression of PPAR-γ, SREBP-1, and SREBP-2 [5, 10–12, 30, 36]. Studies under normobaric hypoxia suggest that SCAP plays a role in modulating the overexpression of SREBP-1 [10–12].

Finally, in the studies reviewed in this chapter, we determined that under both hypobaric and normobaric hypoxia conditions, the expression of PPAR-γ could contribute to the increased synthesis of triglycerides through the activation of acylglycerol-3-phosphate acyltransferase 2 and lipin-1. Additionally, the increase in triglycerides is also driven by the activation of SREBP-1 pathways, which involves the activation of SCD-1 and SCAP. On the other hand, both hypoxic conditions lead to elevated cholesterol levels through increased expression of SREBP-2. The increase in these biomolecules (triglycerides and cholesterol) is crucial in the development of hepatic pathologies such as NAFLD. Notably, HIF-1α is the cornerstone in the activation of both PPAR-γ and SREBPs, which, as previously mentioned, play important roles in the development of hepatic pathologies.

7. Conclusion

Through this review, it was determined that, regardless of the type of hypoxemic exposure, this condition could induce hepatic alterations by increasing the synthesis of triglycerides and cholesterol.

To our knowledge, there is limited information on studies regarding hypobaric hypoxia and its impact on hepatic metabolism. However, both normobaric and hypobaric hypoxia share similarities in the pathways associated with increased synthesis of triglycerides and cholesterol through the overexpression of proteins such as PPAR-γ, SREBP-1, SCD-1, and HMG-CoA. Notably, SREBPs and PPAR-γ are regulated by the stabilization of HIF-1α. Therefore, this review revealed that hypobaric hypoxia could contribute to the development of chronic hepatic pathologies, such as NAFLD. Finally, this chapter facilitates the understanding and identification of key target proteins, including HIF-1, PPAR-γ, SREBP-1, SCD-1, and HMG-CoA reductase, under hypoxic conditions by comparing the effects of hypobaric and normobaric hypoxia on the liver. This finding opens new avenues for research into hepatic pathologies under hypoxic conditions.

Acknowledgements

We would like to thank Patricia Siques and Julio Brito for their support and assistance with this chapter.

Conflict of interest

The authors declare that they have no conflicts of interest.

Author details

Eduardo Pena* and Marco Luza
High-Altitude Medicine Research Center (CEIMA), Arturo Prat University, Iquique, Chile

*Address all correspondence to: eduardopena@unap.cl

References

[1] Grocott MP, Montgomery H, Vercueil A. High-altitude physiology and pathophysiology: Implications and relevance for intensive care medicine. Critical Care. 2007;**11**(1):203. DOI: 10.1186/cc5142

[2] Tremblay JC, Ainslie PN. Global and country-level estimates of human population at high altitude. Proceedings of the National Academy of Sciences of the United States of America. 2021;**118**(18):e2102463118. DOI: 10.1073/pnas.2102463118

[3] Richalet JP, Donoso MV, Jiménez D, et al. Chilean miners commuting from sea level to 4500 m: A prospective study. High Altitude Medicine & Biology. 2002;**3**(2):159-166. DOI: 10.1089/15270290260131894

[4] Osorio J, Siques P, Brito J. Vivir y trabajar en altura. 2nd ed. Iquique, Chile: Fundación Medicina de Altura; 2014

[5] Siques P, Brito J, Naveas N, et al. Plasma and liver lipid profiles in rats exposed to chronic hypobaric hypoxia: Changes in metabolic pathways. High Altitude Medicine & Biology. 2014;**15**(3):388-395. DOI: 10.1089/ham.2013.1134

[6] Zúñiga J, Cancino M, Medina F, et al. N-3 PUFA supplementation triggers PPAR-α activation and PPAR-α/NF-κB interaction: Anti-inflammatory implications in liver ischemia-reperfusion injury. PLoS One. 2011;**6**(12):e28502. DOI: 10.1371/journal.pone.0028502

[7] Chida M, Voelkel NF. Effects of acute and chronic hypoxia on rat lung cyclooxygenase. The American Journal of Physiology. 1996;**270**(5 Pt 1):L872-L878. DOI: 10.1152/ajplung.1996.270.5.L872

[8] Monge C, Leon-Velarde F. El reto Fisiológico de vivir en los Andes. Lima, Peru: Instituto Francés de Estudios Andinos (IFEA), Universidad Peruana Cayetano Heredia (UPCH); 2003. ISBN: 9972-623-27-0

[9] León-Velarde F, Maggiorini M, Reeves JT, et al. Consensus statement on chronic and subacute high altitude diseases. High Altitude Medicine & Biology. 2005;**6**(2):147-157. DOI: 10.1089/ham.2005.6.147

[10] Li J, Bosch-Marce M, Nanayakkara A, et al. Altered metabolic responses to intermittent hypoxia in mice with partial deficiency of hypoxia-inducible factor-1α. Physiological Genomics. 2006;**25**(3):450-457. DOI: 10.1152/physiolgenomics.00293.2005

[11] Li CY, Liu JZ, Wu LP, Li B, Chen LF. Effects of hypobaric hypoxia on adenine nucleotide pools, adenine nucleotide transporter activity and protein expression in rat liver. World Journal of Gastroenterology. 2006;**12**(13):2120-2124. DOI: 10.3748/wjg.v12.i13.2120

[12] Dewi S, Yulhasri Y, Mulyawan W. The impact of intermittent hypobaric hypoxia exposures on triacylglycerol synthesis in rat liver. Reports of Biochemistry And Molecular Biology. 2021;**10**(3):437-444. DOI: 10.52547/rbmb.10.3.437

[13] Savransky V, Nanayakkara A, Li J, et al. Chronic intermittent hypoxia induces atherosclerosis. American Journal of Respiratory and Critical Care Medicine. 2007;**175**(12):1290-1297. DOI: 10.1164/rccm.200612-1771OC

[14] Bhutta BS, Alghoula F, Hypoxia BI, Bruder ED, Lee PC, Raff H. Lipid and fatty acid profiles in the brain, liver,

and stomach contents of neonatal rats: Effects of hypoxia. American Journal of Physiology. Endocrinology and Metabolism. 2005;**288**(2):E314-E320. DOI: 10.1152/ajpendo.00362.2004

[15] Urdampilleta A, González-Muniesa P, Portillo MP, Martínez JA. Usefulness of combining intermittent hypoxia and physical exercise in the treatment of obesity. Journal of Physiology and Biochemistry. 2012;**68**(2):289-304. DOI: 10.1007/s13105-011-0115-1

[16] Beall CM, Strohl KP, Blangero J, et al. Ventilation and hypoxic ventilatory response of Tibetan and Aymara high altitude natives. American Journal of Physical Anthropology. 1997;**104**:427-447. DOI: 10.1002/(SICI)1096-8644(199712)104:4<427::AID-AJPA1>3.0.CO;2-P

[17] Germack R, Leon-Velarde F, De La Barra R, et al. Effect of intermittent hypoxia on cardiovascular function, adrenoceptors and muscarinic receptors in Wistar rats. Experimental Physiology. 2002;**87**(4):453-460. DOI: 10.1111/j.1469-445X.2002.tb00058.x

[18] Sherpa LY, Deji SH, et al. Prevalence of metabolic syndrome and common metabolic components in high altitude farmers and herdsmen at 3700 m in Tibet. High Altitude Medicine & Biology. 2013;**14**(1):37-44. DOI: 10.1089/ham.2012.1051

[19] Gazal S, Espinoza JR, Austerlitz F, et al. The genetic architecture of chronic mountain sickness in Peru. Frontiers in Genetics. 2019;**10**:690. DOI: 10.3389/fgene.2019.00690

[20] Ebner LJA, Samardzija M, Storti F, et al. Transcriptomic analysis of the mouse retina after acute and chronic normobaric and hypobaric hypoxia. Scientific Reports. 2021;**11**(1):16666. DOI: 10.1038/s41598-021-96150-9

[21] Mylonis I, Simos G, Paraskeva E. Hypoxia-inducible factors and the regulation of lipid metabolism. Cells. 2019;**8**(3):214. DOI: 10.3390/cells8030214

[22] Semenza GL. Hypoxia-inducible factor 1 (HIF-1) pathway. Science's STKE. 2007;**2007**(407):cm8. DOI: 10.1126/stke.4072007cm8

[23] Humbert M, Guignabert C, Bonnet S, Dorfmüller P, Klinger JR, Nicolls MR, et al. Pathology and pathobiology of pulmonary hypertension: State of the art and research perspectives. The European Respiratory Journal. 2019;**53**(1):1801887

[24] Ikeda H, Kakeya H. Targeting hypoxia-inducible factor 1 (HIF-1) signaling with natural products toward cancer chemotherapy. Journal of Antibiotics (Tokyo). 2021;**74**(10):687-695. DOI: 10.1038/s41429-021-00451-0. Epub 2021 Jul 30

[25] Ntambi JM. Regulation of stearoyl-CoA desaturase by polyunsaturated fatty acids and cholesterol. Journal of Lipid Research. 1999;**40**(9):1549-1558. DOI: 10.1016/S0022-2275(20)33401-5

[26] Morrison RF, Flier JS. SCD-1 and the regulation of adiposity and insulin sensitivity. The Journal of Clinical Investigation. 2002;**110**(3):289-295. DOI: 10.1172/JCI16111

[27] Yabe D, Yang T, Brown MS. Legitimate roles of sterol regulatory element-binding proteins in lipid metabolism and beyond. The Journal of Clinical Investigation. 2002;**109**(8):1135-1142. DOI: 10.1172/JCI16004

[28] Horton JD, Goldstein JL, Brown MS. SREBPs: Activators of the complete program of cholesterol and fatty acid synthesis in the liver. The Journal of Clinical Investigation.

2002;**109**(9):1125-1131. DOI: 10.1172/JCI16018

[29] Goldstein JL, Brown MS. Regulation of the mevalonate pathway. Nature. 1990;**343**(6257):425-430. DOI: 10.1038/343425a0

[30] Li J, Grigoryev DN, Ye SQ, et al. Chronic intermittent hypoxia upregulates genes of lipid biosynthesis in obese mice. Journal of Applied Physiology. 2005;**99**(5):1643-1648. DOI: 10.1152/japplphysiol.00522.2005

[31] Dolt KS, Karar J, Mishra MK, et al. Transcriptional downregulation of sterol metabolism genes in murine liver exposed to acute hypobaric hypoxia. Biochemical and Biophysical Research Communications. 2007;**354**:148-153

[32] Canouï-Poitrine F, Veerabudun K, Larmignat P, et al. Risk prediction score for severe high altitude illness: A cohort study. PLoS One. 2014;**9**:e100642. DOI: 10.1371/journal.pone.0100642

[33] Richalet JP, Lhuissier FJ. Aging, tolerance to high altitude, and cardiorespiratory response to hypoxia. High Altitude Medicine & Biology. 2015;**16**(2):117-124. DOI: 10.1089/ham.2015.0030

[34] Viscor G, Ricart A, Pagès T, et al. Intermittent hypoxia for obstructive sleep apnea? High Altitude Medicine & Biology. 2014;**15**:520-521. DOI: 10.1089/ham.2014.1060

[35] Lee PC, Jelinek B, Struve M, et al. Effect of hypoxia on metabolic responses in muscle, liver and adipose tissue: Physiological and therapeutic implications. Current Diabetes Reviews. 2021;**17**(6):1002-1010. DOI: 10.2174/1573399817666200713111449

[36] Luo Y, Chen Q, Zou J, Fan J, Li Y, Luo Z. Chronic intermittent hypoxia exposure alternative to exercise alleviates high-fat-diet-induced obesity and fatty liver. International Journal of Molecular Sciences. 2022;**23**(9):5209. DOI: 10.3390/ijms23095209

[37] Li J, Thorne LN, Punjabi NM, et al. Intermittent hypoxia induces hyperlipidemia in lean mice. Circulation Research. 2005;**97**(7):698-706. DOI: 10.1161/01.RES.0000183879.60089.a9

[38] Polotsky VY, Li J, Punjabi NM, Rubin AE, Smith PL, Schwartz AR, et al. Intermittent hypoxia increases insulin resistance in genetically obese mice. The Journal of Physiology. 2003;**552**(1):253-264. DOI: 10.1113/jphysiol.2003.048173

[39] Drager LF, Li J, Shin MK, Reinke C, Aggarwal NR, Jun JC, et al. Intermittent hypoxia inhibits clearance of triglyceride-rich lipoproteins and inactivates adipose lipoprotein lipase in a mouse model of sleep apnoea. European Heart Journal. 2012;**33**(6):783-790. DOI: 10.1093/eurheartj/ehr097

[40] Ntambi J. Regulation of stearoyl-CoA desaturases and role in metabolism. Progress in Lipid Research. 2004;**43**(2):91-104. DOI: 10.1016/S0163-7827(03)00039-0

[41] Foretz M, Pacot C, Dugail I, Lemarchand P, Guichard C, le Lièpvre X, et al. ADD1/SREBP-1c is required in the activation of hepatic lipogenic gene expression by glucose. Molecular and Cellular Biology. 1999;**19**(5):3760-3768. DOI: 10.1128/MCB.19.5.3760

Chapter 6

Hepatoprotective Activity of Proline Derivatives

Vignesh Pandi and Sam Johnson Udhayachandar

Abstract

The liver plays a dynamic role in detoxification, metabolic regulation, and maintaining physiological balance, yet it is highly prone to damage from drugs and toxic substances. Paracetamol overdose is a well-known cause of drug-induced liver injury (DILI), emphasizing the importance of finding effective protective compounds. Proline has shown promise in protecting the liver due to its antioxidant properties and ability to preserve mitochondrial function. This study inspects the liver-protective potential of a synthetic proline-based compound, 1-[(2-hydroxy-anilino) acetyl] pyrrolidine-2-carboxylic acid, through computational and animal model approaches. Molecular docking revealed robust affinity for gamma-glutamyl transpeptidase, a key enzyme in glutathione regulation. Animal studies in rats implied that the compound significantly lowered liver enzyme levels, reduced oxidative stress, and minimized liver tissue damage caused by paracetamol. Additionally, the proline derivative enhances glutamate production, thereby amplifying the glutathione synthesis pathway, further supporting its potential as a hepatoprotective agent.

Keywords: hepatoprotective, gamma-glutamyl transpeptidase, oxidative stress, *In vivo* studies, paracetamol overdose, antioxidant levels, silymarin

1. Introduction

Hepatocytes, the liver's primary cells, are equipped with essential enzymes that support the metabolic functions of processing drugs, neutralizing toxic substances, and eliminating reactive oxygen species (ROS). However, excessive exposure to toxins can surpass the liver's detoxification capacity, resulting in hepatotoxicity. Paracetamol overdose is one of the most common causes of drug-induced liver injury (DILI), contributing significantly to cases of acute liver failure. The toxic byproduct NAPQI accumulates when glutathione (GSH) is depleted or gamma-glutamyl transpeptidase (GGT) is suppressed, causing oxidative stress, mitochondrial dysfunction, and immune disturbances [1].

This research investigates the liver-protective effects of a synthetic proline derivative, 1-[(2-hydroxyanilino) acetyl] pyrrolidine-2-carboxylic acid, using in silico simulations and animal models. It plays a crucial role in supporting the body's homeostasis through detoxification and various metabolic processes.

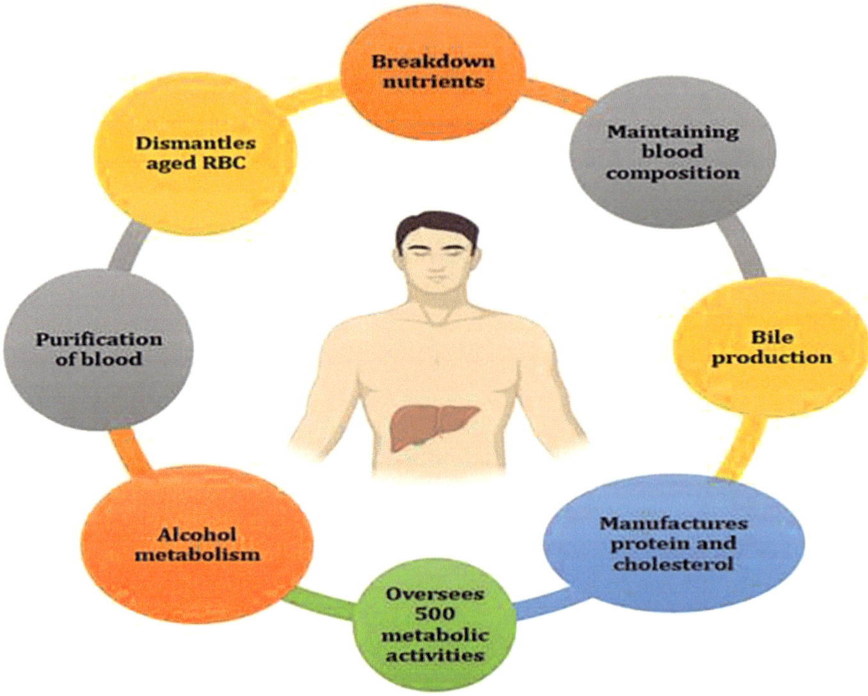

Figure 1.
Functions of the liver.

2. Functions of the liver

The tremendous work of the liver maintains the overall health of the body. It serves as a working factory for protein synthesis for blood plasma, such as albumin and other clotting factors, and glucose regulation by storing it as glycogen. Removing the waste products of drugs, toxins, and RBC, via the bile, and metabolizing the fat by bile production. It processes the nutrients and acts as the storage bag for the vitamins A, D, E, and K. It regulates the chemical composition of blood for proper body function. The overall diagram is illustrated in **Figure 1** [2].

3. Hepatotoxicity

Hepatotoxicity is triggered by the liver's diminished capacity to detoxify and remove hazardous substances as a result of exposure to chemicals, medications, or drugs. More than 900 medications, including NSAIDs, corticosteroids, and anti-tuberculosis medical treatments, are being implicated as potential triggers for drug-induced liver damage (DILI), the main root cause of abrupt liver failure. Oxidative stress, mitochondrial damage, and immunological barrier responses, which are frequently detected by elevated liver enzymes such as ALT, AST, and ALP, are the causes behind DILI. DILI is responsible for over half of all occurrences of acute liver failure and constitutes about 5% of hospital admissions. It is alarming to note that up to 75% of instances of idiosyncratic DILI can culminate in death or liver transplantation.

According to WHO estimates, liver disorders damage almost 29 million people globally each year. Nearly 1 million new incidences of cirrhosis are diagnosed in India each year, making it one of the top 10 causes of fatalities [3].

4. Stages of liver damage

Stage 0: Healthy Liver—The liver is in its normal state with no damage or dysfunction.

Stage 1: Onset of Liver Damage—Early signs of liver injury emerge, often marked by fat buildup or mild inflammation.

Stage 2: Progressing Liver Damage—Liver cells begin to show structural damage, with growing inflammation and scar tissue.

Stage 3: Advanced Liver Damage—Scarring becomes widespread (fibrosis), starting to interfere with liver performance.

Stage 4: Final Stage (Cirrhosis)—Severe and irreversible scarring leads to significant loss of liver function, often progressing to liver failure.

4.1 Causes of hepatotoxicity

Liver damage can be triggered by a wide range of widely used substances, including medications such as acetaminophen, ibuprofen, aspirin, antibiotics like isoniazid and rifampicin, statins, antidepressants, and anticonvulsants. In addition, substances like alcohol, cocaine, heroin, industrial chemicals (e.g., solvents, heavy metals, and pesticides), as well as some herbal products and dietary supplements, also carry the potential to harm the liver.

4.2 Prevention of hepatotoxicity

Early recognition and swift resolution are necessary to minimize hepatotoxicity and reduce the risk of significant liver failure or injury. It is imperative to take prescription medicines exactly as directed and to refrain from taking more than recommended. Patients should be aware of any potential negative effects on the liver and disclose to their physician all substances they consume, including prescription medications, over-the-counter drugs, antioxidants, and herbal products. Limiting or avoiding alcohol consumption is strongly advised. It is essential for individuals who handle hazardous materials to wear protective gear and adhere to safety protocols. The hepatitis A and B vaccinations provide additional protection against liver damage. Healthy lifestyle choices, such as eating a balanced diet, staying active, and maintaining a healthy weight, are crucial for liver health. Moreover, individuals predisposed to liver disease or those undergoing treatments that adversely affect the liver should have regular liver function testing under the supervision of a medical practitioner.

5. Drug toxicity mechanisms

Typically, there are two forms of drug-induced liver toxicity: intrinsic and idiosyncratic. Acetaminophen and carbon tetrachloride are two instances of medications that manifest intrinsic toxicity, which is predictable and dose-dependent and generally originates from the direct adverse consequences of the drug or its metabolites. On the flip side, idiosyncratic toxicity is unpredictable, not dose-dependent, and it is frequently accompanied by relatively rare metabolic reactions in certain people or aberrant immune system reactions [4].

6. Treatment for hepatotoxicity

Recognition and cessation of the toxic substance, constant liver function monitoring, and total abstinence from alcohol and other liver-damaging substances are the first measures in addressing hepatotoxicity. Possible treatments include drugs like diuretics to control fluid buildup, antihistamines for alleviating itching, and ursodeoxycholic acid to enhance bile flow. Advanced interventions like liver transplantation or biopsy may be necessary in catastrophic circumstances. Hepatotoxic agents are generally classified into two categories: metabolism-dependent toxins (e.g., paracetamol, methotrexate, ethanol) and direct-acting toxins (e.g., carbon tetrachloride, cadmium).

7. Glutathione (GSH) and its role

Glutathione (GSH), a tripeptide made up of γ-L-glutamyl-L-cysteinyl glycine, is the most abundant non-protein thiol and plays a key role in detoxification, antioxidant defense, and maintaining redox balance. It is primarily found in the cytosol (80–85%), where it helps neutralize reactive oxygen species (ROS), hydrogen peroxide, and lipid peroxides through the enzyme glutathione peroxidase (GPx). GSH also contributes to the regulation of protein stability and various detoxification processes.

7.1 Glutathione and antioxidant defense

During oxidative stress, glutathione (GSH) is converted to its oxidized form, GSSG, which is then regenerated back to GSH by the enzyme glutathione reductase (GR) using NADPH. In cases of intense oxidative stress, GSSG may either be exported or form mixed disulfides. The GSH-based antioxidant system detoxifies hydrogen peroxide (H_2O_2) through catalase or glutathione peroxidase (GPx) and helps reduce lipid peroxides via glutathione S-transferase (GST), thus playing a crucial role in maintaining redox balance [5].

7.2 Glutathione cycle

The gamma-glutamyl cycle regulates the synthesis, degradation, and recycling of glutathione (GSH), essential for detoxification, redox balance, and amino acid transport. Gamma-glutamyl transpeptidase (GGT) eventually breaks it down into gamma-glutamyl amino acids and cysteinyl glycine, which dipeptidase then breaks down into cysteine and glycine. These amino acids are either converted into other metabolites or delivered to the cell for the manufacturing of proteins. The cycle can be terminated by converting gamma-glutamyl amino acids into 5-oxoproline, which subsequently turns back into glutamate. The modified glutathione cycle (GSH) is deplicted in **Figure 2** [5].

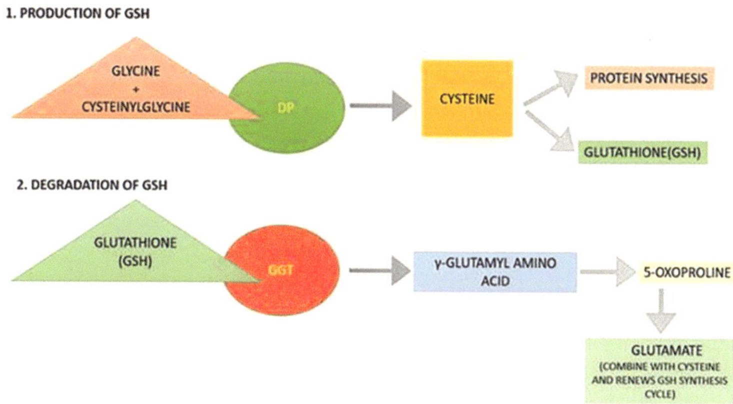

Figure 2.
Glutathione cycle.

8. Hepatoprotective effects of proline

Proline is essential for hepatoprotective functions like immune regulation, hepatic lipogenesis, inflammatory suppressors, and antioxidants.

8.1 Antioxidant defense and liver protection

Proline modulates the liver's antioxidant defense in D-galactosamine-induced hepatitis by enhancing glutathione (GSH) production over 6–12 hours, diminishing reactive oxygen species (ROS) within hours, and accelerating catalase activity. It also emphasizes its hepatoprotective properties by boosting the production of glutathione reductase (GR) and peroxidase (GP), which contribute to conserving mitochondrial function and diminishing liver inflammation.

8.2 Inflammation suppression and liver regeneration

By promoting the IL-6/STAT3 signaling pathway, suppressing TNF-α-induced inflammation, and aiding in liver regeneration, proline promotes survival. By triggering oxidative preconditioning, it raises the liver's ability to withstand stress and destruction, emphasizing its promise as a liver recovery therapy.

8.3 Hepatic lipogenesis and liver function

By elevating the expression of genes such as Fasn, Scd1, and Srebf1, proline promotes the metabolism of liver fat. Because proline has an individual impact on hepatic metabolic activity, it is crucial in the treatment of MASLD and other metabolic liver disorders, in contrast to other amino acids like hydroxyproline or ornithine.

8.4 Immune modulation and liver protection

Hydroxyproline governs immunological responses by hampering autophagy and fostering PD-L1 expression through IFN-γ signaling especially in autoimmune and fibrotic liver diseases.

8.5 Metabolic regulation and liver resilience

Proline oxidase (POX/PRODH) impacts apoptosis, generating ROS, redox harmony, and immune system obstacles signaling by integrating proline metabolism into the TCA cycle. The liver's capacity for enduring stress becomes more efficient, and oxidative phosphorylation is augmented by an impact on HIF-1α pathways.

8.6 Antioxidant and anti-inflammatory properties

Proline administration streamlines oxidative stress, perpetuates GSH levels, and drastically reduces inflammatory markers in bile duct ligation (BDL) mice, which avoids early liver damage. It may help cure cholestatic liver illnesses because it reliably safeguards liver cells from oxidative damage provoked by bile acids, yet shows a slight impact on fibrosis [6].

9. Rationale of the study

Especially in the liver, the gamma-glutamyl cycle serves as crucial for ensuring intracellular GSH levels and redox harmony. This cycle's processing of 5-oxoproline to glutamate is a crucial step because it is crucial to the generation of GSH and antioxidant defense.

This chapter proposes an improved proline derivative that enhances hepatoprotection through a dual mode of action. To spike intracellular glutamate production, the ingredient either acts as a metabolic enhancer or increases 5-oxoprolinase activity. This increases the availability of synthesis substrates for the synthesis of gamma-glutamyl transpeptidase (GGT), an enzyme whose overactivity causes GSH depletion and oxidative stress, which is additionally specifically inhibited by it. This substance provides an all-encompassing approach to lessen oxidative damage in liver illnesses such as drug-induced liver damage (DILI), non-alcoholic fatty liver disease (NAFLD), and cholestatic situations by promoting GSH production and maintaining current GSH stores.

10. Mechanism of paracetamol (APAP) metabolism and hepatotoxicity

A typical medication for pain relief and fever reduction is paracetamol (APAP), however, an overdose can result in abrupt liver failure and drug-induced liver damage (DILI). Because it produces NAPQI, it depletes glutathione (GSH) and causes oxidative stress and damage to liver cells, and it has hepatotoxic effects. Developing successful treatments and enhancing drug safety require a thorough grasp of its toxicity mechanisms and metabolic processes.

11. Metabolism under therapeutic conditions

The liver mostly uses phase II conjugation to metabolize paracetamol at typical dosages. About 33% of paracetamol is broken down by the sulfation pathway, which produces sulfated forms that are excreted by the kidneys.

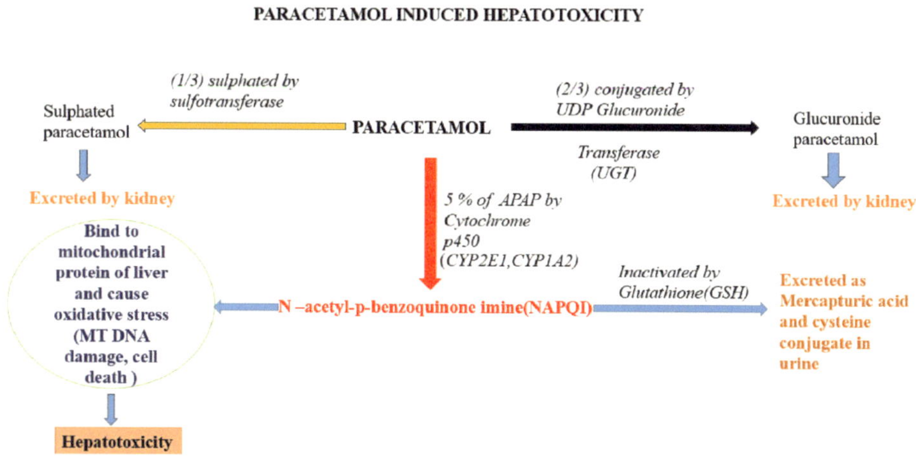

Figure 3.
This graphic highlights the critical role of glutathione in protecting the liver from damage and successfully illustrates the equilibrium between detoxification and detrimental effects in paracetamol metabolism.

UDP-glucuronosyltransferase (UGT) binds the glucuronic acid to paracetamol for excretion during the glucuronidation metabolism, which accounts for around 66% of the total. CYP2E1 and CYP1A2 enzymes metabolize a tiny percentage (about 5%), resulting in NAPQI, a hazardous byproduct that is typically removed by glutathione (GSH). Excess NAPQI causes oxidative stress and liver injury by depleting GSH in overdose cases (**Figure 3**) [7].

11.1 Metabolism under toxic doses/overdose conditions

As a result of the principal detoxification pathways, UGT and SULT, becoming saturated during an overdose of paracetamol (APAP), drug metabolism shifts to CYP enzymes, which produce an excess of the poisonous metabolite NAPQI. When NAPQI builds up, the liver's glutathione (GSH) stores are overloaded and eventually depleted. After that, the unneutralized NAPQI attaches itself to proteins in the mitochondria, causing oxidative stress and ATP depletion, altering mitochondrial function, and raising the generation of oxygen species that are reactive (ROS). The mitochondrial permeability transition (MPT) brought on by these disturbances causes hepatocyte necrosis, which raises the risk of liver failure and causes significant liver damage and inflammation. A clear understanding of this pathway is vital for developing effective hepatoprotective strategies.

12. Drug profile and experimental materials

See **Figure 4** and **Table 1**.

12.1 Materials and methods

Chemicals & Reagents: Silymarin, Paracetamol, Carboxyl Methyl Cellulose, Thiobarbituric Acid, Hepes Buffer, and Sodium Hydroxide (all analytical grade).

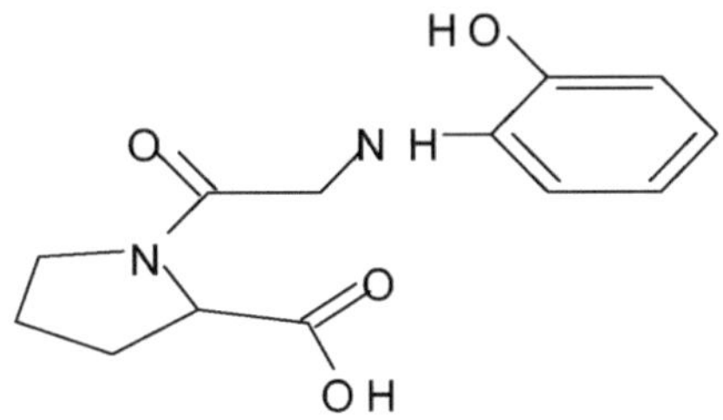

Figure 4.
Structure of 1-[(2-hydroxyanilino) acetyl] pyrrolidine-2-carboxylic acid [8].

IUPAC name	**Pyrrolidine-2-carboxylic acid**
Chemical Formula	C13N2O4H16
Molar mass	264.281 g/mol
Melting point	478–501 k Density: 1.4 g/cm3
Physical Description	Non-essential amino acid exists in the form of crystal
Solubility	1.5 g/100 g
Traditional uses	Skin healing, protein synthesis, antioxidative reaction, Immune response.
Reported activities	Antioxidant properties, Anticonvulsant, Anti-tumor, Anti-diabetic

Table 1.
Drug profile and its properties.

- Diagnostic Kits: AST, ALT, ALP, and LDH (Chemleon Diagnostics).
- Instruments: Centrifuge (Remi), Semi-Auto Analyzer (Agappe MISPA VIVA), pH Meter (ELCO), and UV-Spectrophotometer (Jasco V530).
- Software & Databases: RCSB PDB, Online SMILES Translator, ACD ChemSketch, Schrödinger Maestro, Glide, and QikProp for in silico docking studies.
- Additional Reagents: Anthranilic acid, pyridine, benzoyl chloride, sodium carbonate, ethanol, isatin, paraformaldehyde, hydrazine hydrate, glacial acetic acid, urea, dioxan, and hydroxylamine hydrochloride.
- Additional Instruments: Jasco FT/IR-4100, MR-VIS Visual Melting Range Apparatus, and Elico pH meter.

13. *In silico* studies

Molecular docking was performed to assess the binding affinity of 1-[(2-hydroxyanilino) acetyl] pyrrolidine-2-carboxylic acid with Gamma-glutamyl transpeptidase (GGT, PDB ID: 4Z9O) using Schrödinger's Maestro V12.6 software. Protein and ligand preparation involved energy minimization using the OPLS-3E force field and determining ionization states (pH 6.8–7.2). A receptor grid was created at GGT's active site, and Glide was used to predict binding poses and affinities. ADMET analysis via QikProp evaluated the pharmacokinetic properties and toxicity, while Lipinski's Rule of Five was used to assess the drug-likeness of the compound. This in silico analysis aims to identify proline derivatives with strong GGT binding affinity and favorable pharmacokinetic characteristics.

14. General scheme for the preparation of synthetic derivatives of proline

The synthetic derivatives of 1-[(2-hydroxyanilino) acetyl] pyrrolidine-2-carboxylic acid were synthesized using the following scheme.

14.1 Step A: Preparation of 2-chloro-N-(2-hydroxyphenyl) acetamide

2-Aminophenol (5 g) was mixed with 4 mL chloroacetyl chloride in 30 mL acetic acid and heated for uniform mixing. Sodium acetate trihydrate was added to facilitate product formation. The solid was filtered, dried, and recrystallized in ethanol, yielding 2-chloro-N-(2-hydroxyphenyl) acetamide (**Figure 5**).

14.2 Step B: Preparation of 1-[(2-hydroxyanilino) acetyl] pyrrolidine-2-carboxylic acid

2-chloro-N-(2-hydroxyphenyl) acetamide was dissolved in 30 mL DMF, and 2.5 g potassium carbonate (K_2CO_3) was added. The mixture was stirred for

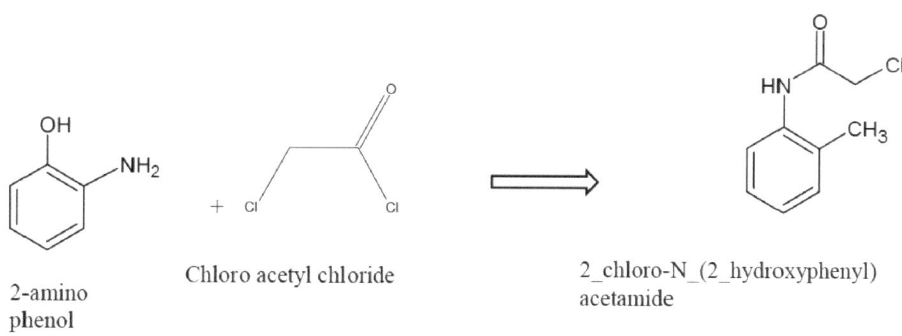

Figure 5.
Preparation of 2-chloro-N-(2-hydroxyphenyl) acetamide.

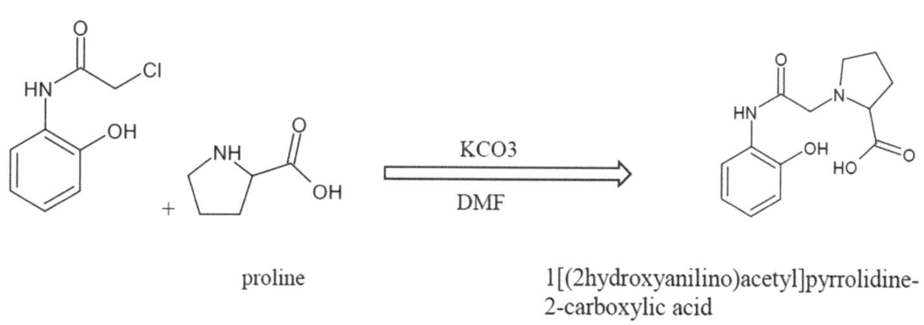

Figure 6.
Preparation of 1-[(2-hydroxyanilino) acetyl] pyrrolidine-2-carboxylic acid.

2.5 hours, followed by the addition of 1.5 g proline, with continued stirring for another 2.5 hours. The solution was extracted with ethanol (3 × 30 mL) using a separatory funnel, and the organic layer was collected, dried, and recrystallized in absolute ethanol, yielding 1-[(2-hydroxyanilino) acetyl] pyrrolidine-2-carboxylic acid (**Figure 6**).

15. Synthesis and characterization

The synthesized compounds were characterized for purity and structural integrity using various techniques. Melting points were determined using MR-VIS and LABINDIA apparatus. Thin Layer Chromatography (TLC) monitored reaction progress, using silica gel and a Benzene: Ethyl acetate (8,2) mobile phase, with spots visualized in an iodine chamber. UV-Vis spectrophotometry (JASCO V-530) analyzed functional groups and purity, while IR spectroscopy confirmed molecular vibrations. NMR spectroscopy (IICB, Kolkata) provided detailed structural elucidation of synthesized proline derivatives (**Figures 7–11** and **Tables 2–4**).

16. *In vivo* studies

16.1 Animal models and ethics

Wistar rats were utilized for hepatotoxicity studies with approval from the IAEC, adhering to CCSEA guidelines. The animals were kept under controlled environmental conditions with free access to food and water, ensuring minimal stress and variability.

Figure 7.
TLC chromatogram of 1-[(2-hydroxyanilino) acetyl] pyrrolidine-2-carboxylic acid.

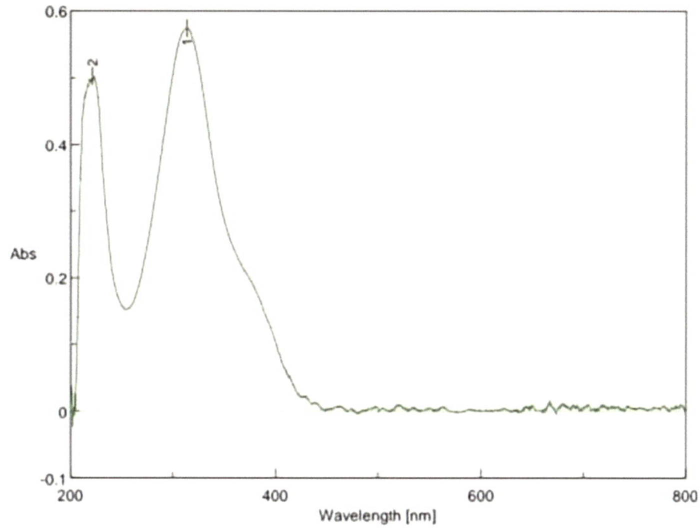

Figure 8.
UV spectrum for 1-[(2-hydroxyanilino) acetyl] pyrrolidine-2-carboxylic acid.

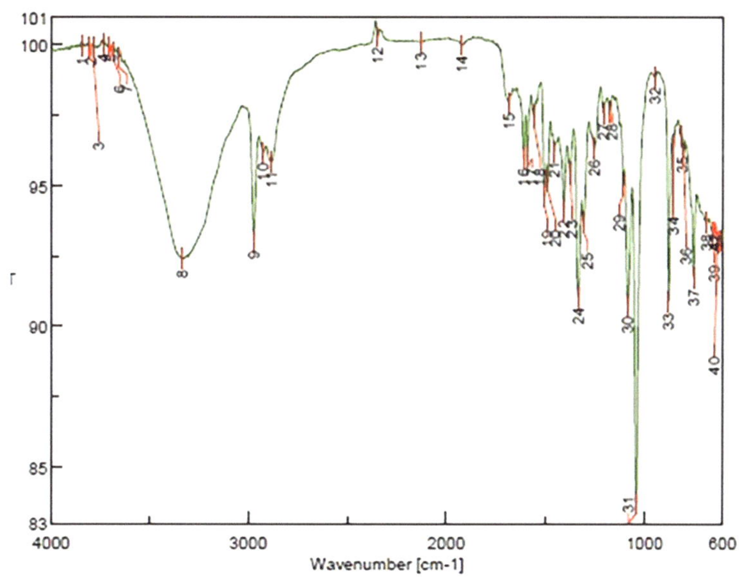

Figure 9.
IR spectrum for 1-[(2-hydroxyanilino) acetyl] pyrrolidine-2-carboxylic acid.

16.2 Acute toxicity studies

Acute oral toxicity was evaluated following OECD guideline 425 (2002) using the "up and down" approach. Female Wistar rats, 8–12 weeks old and weighing between 150 and 200 g, were fasted for 12 hours before being administered escalating doses (55–1750 mg/kg) of the proline derivative. The animals were observed for 14 days to monitor behavioral and physiological responses for safety assessment. Female rats are

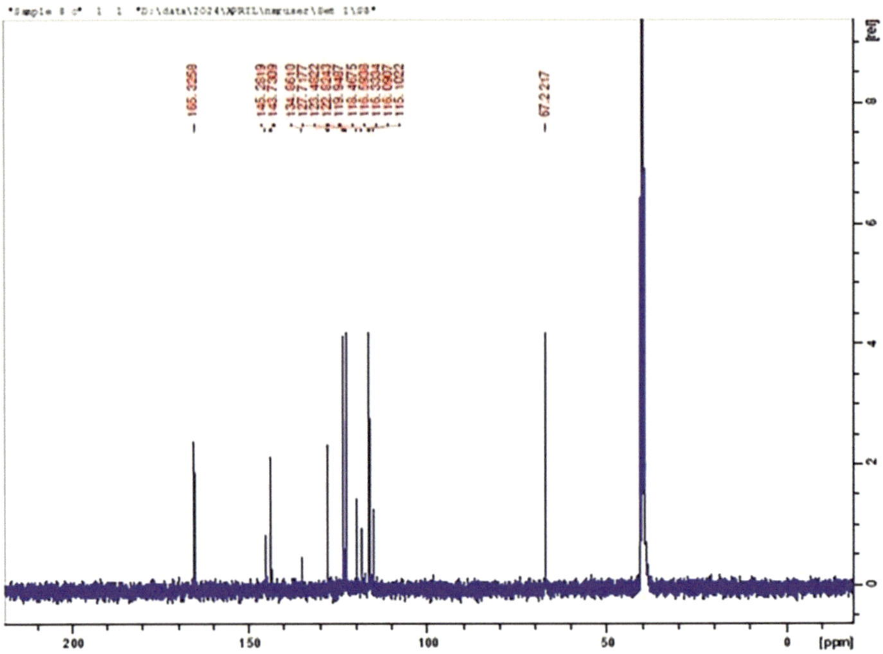

Figure 10.
H^1NMR spectrum for 1-[(2-hydroxyanilino) acetyl] pyrrolidine-2-carboxylic acid.

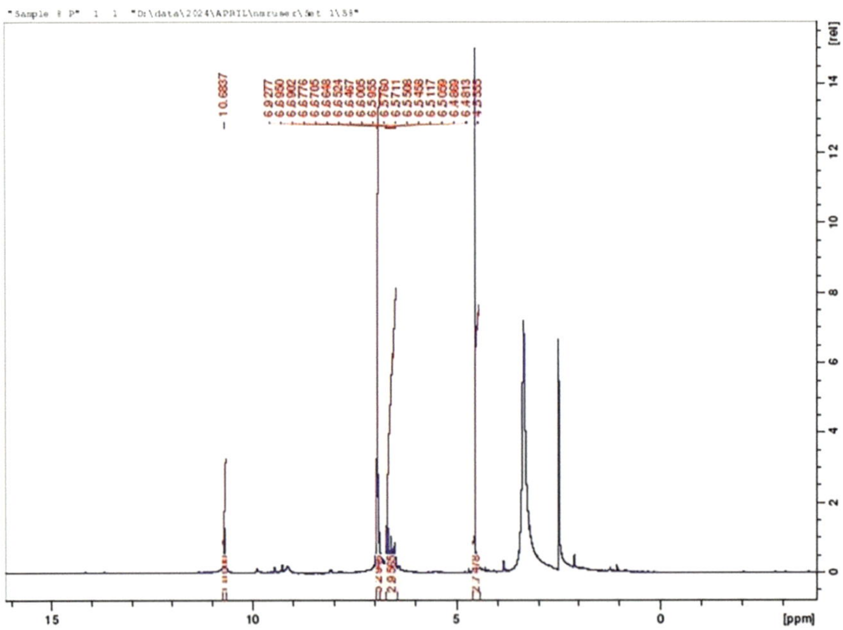

Figure 11.
$C^{13}NMR$ spectrum for 1-[(2-hydroxyanilino) acetyl] pyrrolidine-2-carboxylic acid.

Peak.no	Functional group	Ranges
8	OH-stretching	3470
10,11	NH-stretching	2850
15	C=O- stretching	1600

Table 2.
IR interpretation of 1-[(2-hydroxyanilino) acetyl] pyrrolidine-2-carboxylic acid.

δ ppm	Types of protons
5.29	C-H(Alkene)
6–8.5	Aromatic ring OH
10–13	R COOH

Table 3.
H^1NMR interpretation of 1-[(2-hydroxyanilino) acetyl] pyrrolidine-2-carboxylic acid.

δ ppm	Types of carbon
110–170	CH
165–175	C=O

Table 4.
C^{13}NMR interpretation of 1-[(2-hydroxyanilino) acetyl] pyrrolidine-2-carboxylic acid.

commonly selected for such studies, as outlined in OECD 425, due to their greater sensitivity to toxic effects, which enhances the likelihood of detecting potential toxicity.

17. Paracetamol-induced hepatotoxicity model

Paracetamol-induced hepatotoxicity was established using a single oral dose of paracetamol (2 g/kg). The experiment timeline is 8 days.

Experimental groups were as follows:

Group I: Normal control (normal saline).

Group II: Negative control (paracetamol 2 g/kg).

Group III: Low-dose proline derivative (100 mg/kg).

Group IV: High-dose proline derivative (200 mg/kg).

Group V: Positive control (silymarin 100 mg/kg).

The proline derivative (100, 200 mg/kg)—these doses were chosen to assess dose-dependent efficacy and potential toxicity, and define the therapeutic window, which is the standard approach used in pre-clinical studies. And silymarin was orally administered for 7 days. Paracetamol was administered on Day 7 to induce acute hepatotoxicity following pre-treatment, allowing evaluation of the proline derivative's prophylactic effects. Normal saline was given routinely for 8 days to group I. This design simulates long-term protective treatment and is a validated model for assessing hepatoprotective agents, and animals were euthanized 24 hours later for liver and blood collection.

18. Biochemical and histopathological assessments

Liver function and oxidative stress were assessed using biochemical kits. Serum ALT, AST, and ALP levels indicated hepatocellular damage, while MDA and GSH (Ellman's method) measured oxidative stress and antioxidant capacity. Total protein was quantified via the Lowry method. Histopathology examined hepatocyte degeneration, necrosis, and inflammation.

19. Key findings

Biochemical analysis demonstrated that paracetamol administration significantly increased ALT, AST, ALP, and MDA levels, along with a concomitant reduction in total protein, SOD and GSH levels, confirming hepatocellular injury. Treatment with the proline derivative, particularly at the 200 mg/kg dose, significantly reversed these alterations, restoring biochemical parameters to near-normal levels, comparable to the standard hepatoprotective agent, silymarin (**Tables 5** and **6**).

In contrast, the high-dose proline derivative (200 mg/kg) improved hepatic architecture, similar to silymarin. ANOVA with Dunnett's test confirmed its hepatoprotective efficacy ($p < 0.05$).

20. Histopathological studies

20.1 Effect of SDP 42 on the histopathology of the centrilobular region of liver

Histopathological analysis of liver tissues at 100 and 200 mg/kg doses showed largely preserved architecture with only minor pathological changes, such as mild inflammation, necrosis, or cellular degeneration. Notably, at 200 mg/kg, most lesions were absent compared to the normal control. The overall structural integrity indicates no significant hepatic toxicity and suggests a potential protective effect at the tested doses (**Figure 12**).

21. Discussion and conclusion

This chapter explored the hepatoprotective effects of a novel synthetic proline derivative, 1-[(2-hydroxyanilino) acetyl] pyrrolidine-2-carboxylic acid, against paracetamol-induced liver injury using in silico and in vivo approaches. Molecular docking studies revealed a strong interaction between the compound and gamma-glutamyl transpeptidase (GGT), suggesting its potential role in modulating glutathione (GSH) metabolism. As GGT is essential for maintaining GSH levels, the compound's inhibition of this enzyme may help preserve intracellular GSH and protect liver cells from oxidative damage.

In vivo experiments further confirmed the compound's hepatoprotective effects. Treatment with the derivative significantly reduced liver injury markers such as ALT and AST, lowered oxidative stress indicators like malondialdehyde (MDA), and increased antioxidant levels, including GSH and superoxide dismutase (SOD). Histopathological analysis indicated that the liver tissue retained normal architecture, with decreased levels of necrosis and inflammation compared to the paracetamol-only treated group.

Groups	ALT (U/L)	AST (U/L)	ALP (U/L)	MDA (mmol/min/mg protein)	Total protein (mmol/min/mg protein)
Normal control (Normal saline)	29.35 ± 1.70	82.30 ± 1.97	99.33 ± 4.42	2.61 ± 0.01	512.71 ± 0.89
Negative control (paracetamol)	66.91 ± 2.$_{22}$$^{\#\#\#\#}$	137.83 ± 4.83$^{\#\#\#\#}$	172.11 ± 2.03$^{\#\#\#\#}$	5.90 ± 0.28$^{\#\#\#\#}$	261.80 ± 0.60$^{\#\#\#\#}$
Low-dose SDP (100 mg/kg)	47.46 ± 1.74**	105.43 ± 3.34**	138.86 ± 5.46 ***	4.83 ± 0.17**	371.93 ± 0.73****
High-dose SDP (200 mg/kg)	40.1 ± 1.16****	93.38 ± 3.82****	124.33 ± 3.88****	4.03 ± 0.28****	420.01 ± 0.80****
Standard – silymarin (100 mg/kg)	42.05 ± 1.54****	94.70 ± 3.21****	126.38 ± 3.84****	3.93 ± 0.13****	418.10 ± 0.52****

Values are expressed in Mean ± SEM (n = 6), Data were analysed by One Way ANOVA followed by Dunnett's test. In negative control group, $^{\#\#\#\#}p<0.0001$ compared to normal control. In treatment groups, $^{**}p<0.01$, $^{***}p<0.001$, $^{****}p<0.0001$ compared to negative control.

Table 5.
Effect of SDP on the level of serum biochemical parameters in paracetamol-induced rats.

Groups	SOD (nmoles/min/mg protein)	GSH (nmoles/min/mg protein)
Normal control (Normal saline)	1245 ± 1.28	824.30 ± 1.10
Negative control (paracetamol)	649.90 ± 0.86####	330.25 ± 0.65####
Low-dose SDP (100 mg/kg)	832.50 ± 0.98****	451.05 ± 0.66****
High-dose SDP (200 mg/kg)	933.61 ± 1.03****	554.63 ± 0.96****
Standard silymarin (100 mg/kg)	930.51 ± 0.50****	551.08 ± 0.73****

*Values are expressed in Mean ± SEM (n = 6), Data were analysed by One Way ANOVA followed by Dunnett's test. In negative control group, ####p<0.0001 compared to normal control. In treatment groups, **p<0.01, ***p<0.001, ****p< 0.0001 compared to negative control.*

Table 6.
Effect of synthetic derivative proline on the level of enzymatic and non-enzymatic antioxidants in paracetamol-induced rats.

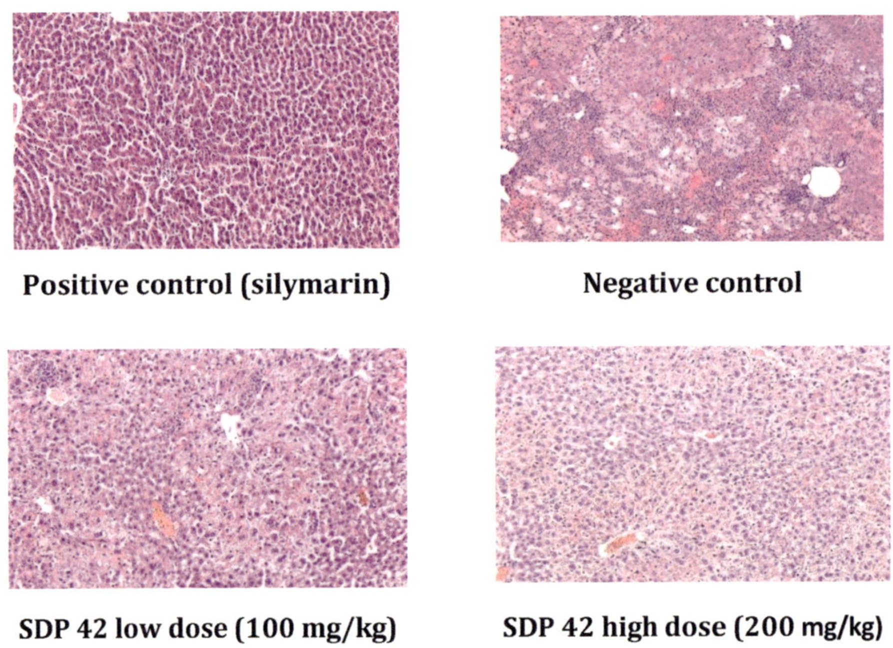

Figure 12.
Histopathological examination of liver sections.

The compound's protective mechanism seems to be twofold: it enhances intracellular glutamate levels, potentially by upregulating 5-oxoprolinase activity or providing metabolic support, which promotes GSH synthesis, and inhibits GGT to prevent GSH degradation [5]. This dual mechanism helps maintain redox balance and reduces oxidative stress, both of which are crucial in preventing liver damage.

This is the first known report of a proline-based derivative that both inhibits GGT and enhances glutamate levels. By targeting multiple steps in the gamma-glutamyl cycle, the compound shows promise as a candidate for the development of hepato-protective drugs. Given its efficacy in the paracetamol-induced liver injury model, it may also be beneficial in treating conditions like drug-induced liver injury (DILI), non-alcoholic fatty liver disease (NAFLD), and cholestasis.

In conclusion, the positive results from both computational and experimental studies suggest that this compound has significant therapeutic potential, warranting further investigation into its pharmacological efficacy and safety for clinical application in liver diseases.

Acknowledgements

I extend my sincere gratitude to my mentor, Dr. K. Asok Kumar, for his moral guidance and valuable suggestions throughout my work. I also thank Dr. M. Uma Maheswari for her constant support and encouragement. Special thanks to my colleague Athira Pankajakshan and Giridharan for their help and cooperation. I am deeply grateful to my family and friends for their unwavering support and patience. Lastly, I appreciate the support of the teaching and non-teaching staff of the College of Pharmacy, SRIPMS, Coimbatore.

Declaration

All the content and research work have been written and developed by me. I confirm that the book does not infringe on any copyrights or legal agreements. Full credits were given for the external source and references.

I confirm that this book has not been copied from any other sources. This is completely based on my research work.

Abbreviations

ADH	alcohol dehydrogenase
ALP	alkaline phosphatase
ALT	alanine transaminase
AST	aspartate aminotransferase
BDL	bile duct ligation
CCSEA	committee for control and supervision of experiments on animals
CYP	cytochrome P
OECD	the organization for economic co-operation and development
GSH	glutathione
GGT	gamma-glutamyl transferase
GP	glutathione peroxidase
GPx	glutathione peroxidase
GSSG	Glutathione disulfide
H1 NMR	proton nuclear magnetic resonance
IAEC	institutional animal ethics committee
IR	infrared
PDB	protein data bank
POX	proline oxidase
PRODH	proline dehydrogenase
ATP	adenosine triphosphate

ALT	alanine transaminase
ALP	alkaline phosphatase
NSAIDs	non-steroidal anti-inflammatory drugs
NAPQI	N-acetyl-p-benzoquinone imine
TNFα	tumor necrosis factor alpha
ADMET	absorption, distribution, metabolism, excretion, and toxicity
NADPH	nicotinamide adenine dinucleotide phosphate hydrogen

Author details

Vignesh Pandi[1] and Sam Johnson Udhayachandar[2*]

1 JSS College of Pharmacy, JSS Academy of Higher Education and Research, Ooty, The Nilgiris, Tamil Nadu, India

2 Sri Ramakrishna Institute of Paramedical Sciences, Coimbatore, India

*Address all correspondence to: mail2samjohnson@gmail.com

References

[1] Arias IM et al. The Liver: Biology and Pathobiology. 6th ed. Wiley; 2020. Available from: https://www.wiley.com/en-us/The+Liver%3A+Biology+and+Pathobiology%2C+6th+Edition-p-9781119436829 [Accessed: February 20, 2025]

[2] Kalra A, Yetiskul E, Wehrle CJ, Tuma F. Physiology, liver. In: StatPearls [Internet]. 2023. Available from: https://www.ncbi.nlm.nih.gov/books/NBK535438/ [Accessed: July 1, 2025]

[3] Meharie BG, Amare GG, Belayneh YM. Evaluation of hepatoprotective activity of the crude extract and solvent fractions of *Clutia abyssinica* (*Euphorbiaceae*) leaf against CCl_4-induced hepatotoxicity in mice. Journal of Experimental Pharmacology. 2020;**12**:137-150

[4] Kaplowitz N. Idiosyncratic drug hepatotoxicity. Nature Reviews. Drug Discovery. 2005;**4**(6):489-499

[5] Lu SC. Glutathione synthesis. Biochimica et Biophysica Acta (BBA) - General Subjects. 2013;**1830**(5):3143-3153

[6] Heidari R, Mohammadi H, Ghanbarinejad V, Ahmadi A, Ommati MM, Niknahad H, et al. Proline supplementation mitigates the early stage of liver injury in bile duct ligated rats. Journal of Basic and Clinical Physiology and Pharmacology. 2018;**30**(1):91-101

[7] Hinson JA, Roberts DW, James LP. Mechanisms of acetaminophen-induced liver necrosis. Handbook of Experimental Pharmacology. 2010;(196):369-405. DOI: 10.1007/978-3-642-00663-0_12

[8] Pyrrolidine-2-carboxylic acid;(2S)-pyrrolidine-2-carboxylic acid|C10H18N2O4|CID 66777928 - PubChem [Internet]. Available from: https://pubchem.ncbi.nlm.nih.gov/compound/66777928 [Accessed: July 1, 2025]